# BONDS
## *of*
# LOVE

# SARAH K

HARPER

This book is a work of non-fiction based on the author's experiences.
In order to protect privacy, names, identifying characteristics, dialogue,
location and details have been changed or reconstructed.

## HARPER

An imprint of HarperCollins*Publishers*
77–85 Fulham Palace Road,
Hammersmith, London W6 8JB

www.harpercollins.co.uk

First published by HarperCollins*Publishers* 2013

1 3 5 7 9 10 8 6 4 2

A catalogue record for this book is
available from the British Library

ISBN: 978-0-00-723767-8

Printed and bound in Great Britain by
Clays Ltd, St Ives plc

**MIX**
Paper from
responsible sources
**FSC** **FSC® C007454**

FSC™ is a non-profit international organisation established to promote
the responsible management of the world's forests. Products carrying the
FSC label are independently certified to assure consumers that they come
from forests that are managed to meet the social, economic and
ecological needs of present and future generations,
and other controlled sources.

Find out more about HarperCollins and the environment at
**www.harpercollins.co.uk/green**

# Chapter One

Even with the blindfold on I knew without a shadow of a doubt that it was Max. There was no mistaking him. It couldn't be anyone else. I recognised the way he moved around me, the sound of his breathing and the scent of his aftershave – a subtle blend of sandalwood and musk that was so familiar it made my mouth water.

I knew him so well that I could practically feel him, and I knew that, whatever happened, with Max there I would be safe and that we would have a good time. More than a good time – we'd have a great time.

I smiled. My sense of relief was mixed with anticipation and an unexpected ache in my heart. Up until that moment I hadn't realised just how much I had missed him. It had been too long.

He moved in closer and whispered my name, tracing my lips with a single finger. The sound of his voice brought tears to my eyes. I wanted to say something to him, but I knew the rules. Submissives only speak when they are spoken to or given permission to speak. Whispering my name was no permission at all.

A cool breeze made me shiver. Behind the blindfold I closed my eyes and drank in Max's touch. He was an expert when it came to knowing how and where to touch me. My pulse quickened as his fingers moved on, stroking my jaw, outlining the curve of my ear, sliding up into my hair. At first it was just the lightest of touches, so delicate that it made my skin tingle, but I knew Max. There would be more. There was always more with Max. His particular gift was the way he could combine pain with pleasure and still have me begging for more. His fingers tightened, twisting my hair into a firm knot, making me gasp as he pulled me close up against him.

'I've missed you, Sarah,' he murmured.

I could feel his breath on my skin and the heat of his body as he cupped my breast with his other hand, caressing the nipple that hardened under his touch, his long nimble fingers teasing and pinching it, making me moan with pleasure and increasing my anticipation of what might follow. My whole body was responding to him, coming alive under his caress. I could feel the desire rising from somewhere deep inside me. I wanted Max so much – it felt like forever since we had been together. I moaned softly, letting go, surrendering to him.

Max murmured his approval and whispered words of endearment as his hand moved lower, down over my ribs, brushing my hips and moving down across my stomach, working its way down over the rise of my sex and sliding unhindered between my legs.

God, this was wonderful. I threw back my head and gasped as he stroked me, his touch at its most tender and knowing, caressing me, making me writhe with pure pleasure. It was the sweetest torture as he explored the soft folds of my sex. I let out a little sob of pleasure as his fingertips finally found my clitoris.

As his fingers found their rhythm I leaned against him, relishing the sensation of his strong muscular body, moaning with sheer delight, feeling every caress, every knowing touch, feeling the pleasure intensify, building and building, bringing me closer and closer to the edge. Finally I cried out and, unable to hold back and breaking all the rules, called out his name.

Even before the sound was out I was instantly awake, torn from sleep, denied the impending climax. I found myself sitting bolt upright in bed, cold and shocked and trembling like a leaf. I looked round, trying to get my bearings. The room was empty, the only light came from the street lamp across the road, throwing a jaundiced yellow stripe across the bedroom floor.

The images and sensations had been so vivid that for a moment I couldn't believe I'd imagined them. I felt like I'd been robbed and reached out in the darkness, a part of me still convinced that Max might be there somewhere, despite knowing that I had only dreamed him. Unsurprisingly, all that was there was darkness, the only sound the tick-tick-tick of my bedroom clock. I stretched out further, feeling my way across the bed, but it was cold and empty.

I lay there for a while thinking about him and trying to get back to sleep, snuggling down under the duvet, trying to relax, but it was impossible. The harder I tried the more awake I felt. Eventually I gave up, switched on the bedside lamp, pulled on a robe and went downstairs to make some tea and try to clear my head.

Max and I had split up months ago, but this was the first time since then that I had dreamed about him and certainly the first time I'd ever been so aroused while sleeping. I could still feel the dull ache of unsatisfied longing, still there, low down in my belly.

I'm a writer, and alongside romantic novels I've written erotic fiction for years, including lots about BDSM (bondage, discipline, sadism and masochism), but after a lifetime of fantasy it had been Max who had finally taken me by the hand and introduced me to the real-life delights of being a submissive. My relationship with Max had been a steep learning curve. He was a Dom (BDSM shorthand for the dominant partner) and under his guidance I had finally found a safe place to explore the submissive fantasies that had haunted me all my adult life.

I'd spent half a lifetime thinking about and then finally writing about the world of BDSM without so much as stepping over the threshold – until I met Max, that is. Fresh out of a marriage, I had decided that it was now or never and had put an ad on a BDSM website. Over the course of several weeks I'd met lots of men who were keen to help me explore my sexually submissive ideas, but in the end it was Max I chose as my first ever real-life Master, and, even though our relationship was over and had been for months, there was a part of me that still loved him.

Under his tutelage I had explored a whole new world of delight, of pleasure and pain and fun, and discovered a level of intimacy that I had never experienced inside a vanilla relationship. Even though it was me who had finally called it a day, Max was going to be a very hard act to follow. He had been a friend and lover as well as a Master. The truth was, I missed him. A lot.

Since he and I had split up I'd been window-shopping on some of the mainstream dating websites as well as the BDSM ones, but I hadn't felt inspired to post a profile – as I said, Max was going to be a hard act to follow. So instead I hunkered down and got on with the business of being single, not feeling quite ready or emotionally robust enough to launch myself back out onto the dating scene, not really having the energy or the inclination to start over – until now, that is. Because the day after dreaming of Max was the day I'd arranged to have my first date with another potential Dom. I couldn't help wondering if that was what had sparked the dream in the first place.

Finding any new relationship is tough enough without the added pressure of finding a man you would trust enough to tie you up. I had been persuading myself that maybe Max was a one-off, a mad fling, a crazy notion. The problem was: what came next? Where did I go from there? Was there a way back to normal?

When we first started seeing each other, Max had warned me even before we started our relationship that going back to straight sex and a vanilla relationship after tasting the delights of BDSM and the intensely intimate connection between Master and submissive was close to impossible.

So there I'd been, still smarting from splitting up with Max, unable or more accurately unwilling to go back to him and not quite ready to go forward, when the phone rang.

I'd been working in my office on a new book. The caller display read 'number withheld'. I wondered if it might be Gabbie, one of my best and oldest friends, and also regularly single. I'd left her a voicemail suggesting that it was high time we got together and had a girls' night in or out, and I promised not to cry as long as she promised not to give every man in the bar a score out of ten, so I was surprised when a male voice said, 'Hi, is that Sarah?'

I hesitated. 'Yes, it is. Who's speaking?'

'I don't know if you remember me. My name's Alex. We spoke a while back about your ad.'

'We did? What ad?' I was racking my brains. It had been a long time since I'd put an ad on any of the straight or BDSM dating websites, and I'd never advertised anything anywhere else.

'Oh, I'm sorry. Maybe I've got the wrong number. It was a while ago now. You were looking for a Dom.'

'And we spoke?' I said cautiously. I had taken down my personal ad when I'd started seeing Max regularly and, as I said, I hadn't felt anywhere near ready to put it back up on the site since we split up, so if Alex was right we'd spoken a long, *long* time ago.

'Only very briefly,' Alex said. 'You were just off to meet someone and said you didn't think it was fair to talk to me until you'd met him. Anyway, I was going through my inbox just now, saw your name and thought I'd give you a ring.' He laughed. 'Nothing ventured ...'

While he was talking I opened my email and typed 'Alex' into the search engine to see if I could find his original mail.

'To be perfectly honest I'm not really looking at the moment,' I said, eyes working down the list of names. His name wasn't there, although that didn't necessarily mean anything; after meeting Max I had deleted most if not all of the other contenders, so it wasn't all that surprising.

'Bad experience?' asked Alex. It was interesting that he didn't assume I was living happily ever after in nipple clamps and handcuffs.

'No, not at all. Just —' I felt around for the right words. How did you explain a fragile, needy ex-girlfriend with a child and a good man with a big heart desperately trying to do the right thing by everyone involved? It was a long story and certainly not one I intended to go into during the first phone call with someone I didn't know.

'Complicated?' Alex suggested.

'Kind of, yes,' I said, wondering why I didn't just hang up.

'Me too. I was chatting to this woman online for a couple of months, Annabel. She sounded perfect. Anyway, we arranged to meet, and it turned out she was a bloke, Archie — fourteen stone, five feet two, buck teeth and —'

He caught me completely off-guard and I laughed. 'You're joking.'

Alex laughed too. 'Yes, actually, I am, but not completely. I started seeing someone and I discovered pretty quickly that she was married and just looking for a bit of kinky fun on the side, which is not what I'm looking for. I was wondering, how about we meet up for lunch and swap horror stories?'

Now it was my turn to laugh again. 'That's a bit of a leap.'

'True, but not that much, and I'm not a stalker or a loony. I've been divorced four years and I've spent a lifetime thinking about this. And I'm a newbie too, so it would be good to talk to someone who is looking for the same thing, wouldn't it?'

'Which is what?'

'True love, world peace and to be able to play the guitar like Ry Cooder?'

'I'm not sure about world peace,' I said, amused and charmed and almost convinced.

'Okay. So how about you tell me some more about yourself,' Alex said.

'Haven't we already done this?' I asked.

'Probably, but it was a long time ago now. I've probably forgotten all the interesting bits. How about we do it again. Do you like fish?'

'What?' I'm sure if he had asked me that before I would have remembered. 'Is this one of your standard getting-to-know-you questions?'

'No.' He laughed. 'It's just that I've got a friend who runs this great little seafood restaurant down on the coast. I was thinking that we could maybe meet there, have a nice lunch, interview each other, decide it was all a horrible mistake and head home older but wiser. What do you think?' He told me the place he meant and I Googled it as we spoke. It wasn't that far from me and maybe, I reasoned, getting out and about would do me good, help me heal the big painful scar that splitting up

with Max had left. If nothing else, once I had decided
he was a total no-no, I could always take a walk on
the beach.

'We could road test the new season's menu,' Alex was
saying. 'They do a really good sharing platter.'

'And you need someone to share with?' I suggested.

'Got it in one.' I liked the sound of his voice. But there
was a part of me that had been thinking that the last thing
I needed right now was another man in my life. I was still
feeling mangled. I'd already thought maybe it was time to
kick back, take time out, give up on men and get some
cats. It seemed a lot more appealing than getting my heart
broken all over again.

'I'm not sure –' I began.

Alex laughed. 'No, me neither. How about we just give
it a go? I promise not to be weird,' he said.

I hesitated. Oh, what the hell. It was ages since I had
been out with a man, ages since I'd been anywhere actually. 'Okay,' I said. 'But the first hint of weirdness and I'm
out of there.'

'Good call,' said Alex. 'When do you fancy meeting up?
Are you free this weekend?'

'This weekend?'

'Too soon?'

'No, no, I'm happy to meet up.' What I meant was that
I was happy to meet up and get it over with. First time
around it had taken me dozens of coffees, dates and lunches
with would-be Doms before I met Max.

For me, as with any relationship, there has to be some
kind of attraction there, some kind of chemistry between

9

a Dom and a sub, and you don't know if it's there until you actually meet someone face to face. Even getting along well on the phone is really no guarantee that that magic *something* is there.

First time around with online dating, both with vanilla and BDSM, I'd realised very early on that if you don't meet someone fairly quickly you run the risk of making whoever you are talking to into whatever it is you are looking for, filling in the gaps with your imagination, expectations and hopes. It's always much, much better to meet any hopefuls quickly rather than be desperately disappointed later.

And if my previous experiences of online dating were anything to go by, the likelihood of Alex being *the one* or of us having that immediate chemistry were close to zero, but it would be good to go out, have a nice meal, meet someone new and get on to the next bit of the healing process. Maybe I should see meeting Alex as a good practice run, a way of getting back up on the horse.

So, while Alex chatted, I went through the motions of opening my diary and flicking through the pages, giving myself time to think, wondering whether I really was ready to start over.

Did I really want a relationship based on BDSM? Did I want to play again? The truthful answer was yes, and unless I planned to spend the rest of my life alone I had to get out there. There was no way I was going to find a relationship – BDSM or otherwise – by running scared and hiding away in my office, so meeting up with Alex seemed as good a place to start as any.

'How about Sunday?' I suggested, in a tone that I hoped implied I might just be able to squeeze him into my hectic social calendar.

'Great. Sunday's fine,' Alex said. 'Shall we say one o'clock?'

'Okay.'

'I've still got your email address here. I'll book us a table with a sea view and email you a map.'

'Okay, sounds like a plan.'

He laughed. 'So far, so good. Do you want me to hang up now?' he asked.

'Maybe, unless you've got something interesting to say, or are you saving that for Sunday?'

'Oh, very sharp,' he said, aping a wince. 'I'll go. I don't want to use up all my best lines.'

'Alex, wait,' I said hastily. I had no idea who he was or what he was into and couldn't, truth be told, ever remember talking to him before.

'What is it?' he asked.

'Would you mind sending me your profile again? I don't think I kept it,' I said, hoping that he wouldn't be offended.

'Of course I can.' And this time the laughter was even louder. 'Good job I'm thick-skinned, isn't it?' he said. Seconds later his profile dropped into my inbox.

And so, after the dream about Max had woken me, it was Alex's profile that I was reading while sitting in my kitchen, cradling a mug of tea, at three o'clock in the morning with my laptop open on the table, trying very,

very hard to get Max out my mind. I hadn't consciously thought about him for weeks and had resisted the temptation to ring, text or email him. The problem was that Max had been my passport into another world, one I had thought about for years and, against my better judgement and good sense, I had fallen for him hard and fast. I'd expected quite a lot of things from BDSM, but falling in love really hadn't been one of them.

Looking at it now in the cool, clear light of dawn, I wasn't sure if it was because of who Max was or what he had offered me. One thing was for sure; I was very determined to take it a lot slower next time. It wasn't that love wasn't on the agenda, it was just that this time I'd be more cautious.

But love or no love, meeting Max had had a profound effect on me. Oddly enough, exploring submission in my private life had helped me feel far more confident and at ease with myself in my normal everyday life, as if by being at ease with my sexuality I had finally come home to who I truly was. It felt good, as if all sorts of dispiriting thoughts and feelings inside my head had finally fallen into place.

Among other things, Max had given me the confidence to let go, to enjoy our sexual encounters as a game, a rich complex role-play where a person could explore all of who they were – and with the right person it could be as heady as any drug. That night's dream had come as a complete revelation, it had seemed so vivid and painfully real. I was obviously missing him, and the sexual satisfaction that he brought me, much more than I had realised. If I closed my eyes I could still feel the brush of Max's fingertips on my flesh.

I made an effort to turn my attention back to the screen of my laptop and to Alex's online profile. It said that he was six feet tall, blond, a divorcee in his late forties with grown-up children and his own home. He listed things he liked out in the real world and those he wanted to explore in the BDSM world. Ropes and gags and blindfolds: a list of things that excited me and also made me slightly nervous, all neatly laid out in a little table of preferences. Alongside what he liked or wanted to try, Alex had listed his hard limits, which were pretty standard: no blood, no blades, no needles, no breath-play, no minors and nothing between him and any partner that wasn't consensual. Sane, safe and consensual. One of the mantras of BDSM play.

He also said he was respectful of any limits, pain threshold, likes and dislikes, although like most Doms he'd try to push the boundaries sometimes, but would honour an agreed safe word that when spoken would stop play immediately. Apparently he had no hang-ups, and in a perfect world was looking for a real relationship that had BDSM at its core. It sounded like the idea I had been toying with – a real-life relationship, but with a BDSM twist that would flavour any encounters and spice up the physical side of things.

Which brought me right back to Max, who had said that sustaining a long-term relationship that could encompass both was close to impossible. A good Dom and sub relationship was based on respect, a sense of formality and a slight distance. What respect would I have for my Dom if we were over-familiar, if I saw him stretched out on the sofa in tracksuit bottoms or had to try to persuade him to take the bins out? Familiarity, Max had argued, really did breed contempt and destroyed the Dom-sub dynamic.

It was this that, despite loving the thrill of submission and enjoying our time together, had given me mixed feelings about Max and how long we could last as a couple. He had told me early on that he was looking for a relationship where the role-play never ended. While we were together he would always be the Dom and I, his partner, the sub – whatever happened, wherever we were, there would be no let up, no time off; we would always be in role.

True, sometimes the atmosphere was lighter, sometimes more intense, but the bottom line was that Max didn't want the easy familiarity of everyday life with a partner so much as the charge, the thrill of the heady sexual and social encounters that the BDSM lifestyle brought him. More to the point, for Max BDSM was the only truly satisfying way for him to enjoy a sexual relationship. He found vanilla sex dull and unsatisfying.

Even when I was with him – and we had some fabulous times – I was always concerned, because I knew without a shadow of a doubt that, much as I loved it, I couldn't live full time within a strict BDSM relationship. I wasn't sure anyone could, but what had rapidly become apparent to me was that, while I did need, like and enjoy that Dom-sub dynamic, in an ideal world what I wanted was someone who could play and then slip back into normal life. It was a big, big ask.

Reading Alex's profile, looking at what he liked and enjoyed, it was all pretty standard stuff. There was certainly nothing on there that set alarm bells ringing. Unusually, Alex had also sent a full-face photo, and he looked okay – more than okay. He had a rugged, nicely made face, with a strong jawline and big blue eyes. In a second photo he had sent he looked as if he might be on holiday. He was casually dressed and standing in a bar, with the people around him carefully cropped out and pixelated. What did shine through from both the photographs and his profile was a sense of warmth and good humour. The way he wrote was bright and intelligent, and the profile was carefully put together.

So, I knew what Alex looked like, he didn't sound like a loony, he sounded like he might be good company and I was happy to be going; so why the dream about Max? I glanced outside into the grey light of the new day trying to analyse it. Unfinished business maybe? One last fond look at what might have been? I wasn't sure, but I did know that it was too early to be up worrying about what had happened in the past and what the future might hold. I couldn't go back to what I had with Max, I had to move on, and meeting Alex was the first step. The sooner I took it, the sooner I could get on with the rest of my life. So I switched off my laptop and headed back upstairs to bed. Within moments of slipping beneath the duvet I dropped into a deep, dreamless sleep.

# Chapter Two

The restaurant was closed. It said so on a large blackboard that had been propped up against the wall outside the car park. I'd been so focused on the road and how to get to the place where we were meeting that the sign took me completely by surprise, so – mid-turn – I carried on turning and sailed into the car park, where a red-and-white striped barrier had been erected across the parking spaces and a small group of men with a van, high-visibility vests and hard hats were all gathered around what looked like a freshly dug hole outside the main entrance to the restaurant.

The main building was long and low with dormer windows set into the swooping roof, and it turned back on itself to enclose a little paved courtyard with tables and benches that caught the mid-morning sun. It would have been the perfect spot for lunch – if it had been open.

As I pulled to a halt another car pulled up alongside mine. Looking across at the driver I realised that it was Alex, who waved and smiled back at me and then rolled down his window.

'Hi there. You found it all right then?' he said, his face broadening into a smile. If anything he looked better than he had in his photo, which was a pleasant surprise. He was lightly tanned, with tousled sun-bleached hair and vibrant blue eyes.

I nodded. 'Yes, thanks,' I said. 'And so did the water authority by the looks of it. Did you invite them?'

Alex laughed. 'Bloody gatecrashers. It looks serious though. I'm thinking we might have to have a change of venue. If you want to wait here, I'll just go and see what's going on.' He climbed out of his car, locked it and headed over towards the restaurant.

Being naturally nosey I got out and followed him. Alex was taller than I'd expected – don't get me started on how many men lie about their height on online dating sites – and he was well built, with broad shoulders and long legs. He was wearing a blue-and-white checked open-neck shirt under a charcoal-grey jacket, with faded Levis and nice shoes, and so far was exactly as advertised in his profile. As we got to the barriers, he paused.

'Nice to meet you, by the way,' he said. There was something quite boyish about him, and although he wasn't classically handsome he was nice looking, with a broad, generous mouth and very naughty eyes. I made myself take a calm, collected step back from all the approving noises my brain was making; we were playing it cool, remember? Slowly, slowly this time. I extended a hand. Alex shook it and as he did we both made a slightly awkward manoeuvre and then stepped closer, at which point he kissed me on the cheek.

'This isn't going quite how I planned,' he added.

'Well, that's good. If you're going to arrange some excitement I'd rather it didn't involve –' I was about to say a water leak when I got a whiff of whatever it was that was lurking in the bottom of the hole. 'God, that smells awful.'

He laughed. 'Anyway, I'm Alex. It's nice to meet you at long last.'

'Sarah,' I said.

His grip was warm and firm and his hand so big that it swallowed mine whole. 'Delighted, and you know you look just like your photo.'

'Which is rare,' I said ruefully.

He nodded. 'You can say that again.'

'You too. So far, so good.'

He grinned. 'I think so.'

I had sent him a photo in response to his; I wanted Alex to recognise me when we met and also know what he was letting himself in for. Although I'm not overweight, I am a proper grown-up woman with curves and wrinkles, not a smooth stick insect. Lots of the men on both BDSM and ordinary websites are looking for women much younger than themselves, which is fine, but unless they're in their dotage, I'm not one of them. Alex, who was in his mid-forties, had specified that he wanted to meet someone within three to five years of his age, which was also rare and suggested he was looking for something more than just the physical – well, I hoped that was what it meant.

He eased one of the barriers to one side. 'I'm just going to nip inside and see if I can see –' But before he could complete the sentence, a man in chef's whites appeared from one of the service doors of the restaurant and hurried towards us, waving madly and grinning like a loon. Alex waved back.

'No need, here he comes. This is the friend I was telling you about. His name's Cash,' Alex said. 'And this place is his new baby. He and his partner bought it last year. They haven't been open that long. I hope this water thing isn't anything too serious. They've put every penny they've got into this place.'

'Hello,' said Cash, looking from face to face.

'Bit extreme, isn't it? Trying to keep us out, are you?' said Alex to Cash, nodding towards the barriers.

'We do our best to try and keep the riff-raff out,' said the man, and then he slipped through a gap in the barriers and they embraced and slapped each other on the back in the way that men do. 'I'm so sorry, mate. I did ring to try and let you know. It's some sort of leak. We've had to close until they fix it. I left you a message first thing this morning but presumably you were too busy to pick it up.' As he spoke, Cash smiled in my direction.

Following his gaze, Alex did the introductions. 'Cash, this is Sarah, Sarah this is Cash. We go back years; Cash and I were at school together.'

'Many moons ago now,' said the man, taking my hand and pressing it to his lips. 'Delighted to meet you. Any friend of Alex's –'

Alex raised his eyebrows. 'Don't mind Cash, he always was a lech.'

Cash grinned. 'I'm just so sorry that I can't offer you lunch.'

'Me too. Do they know what the problem is?' asked Alex, glancing over towards the posse of workmen. 'I hope it's nothing serious.'

'Me too. I'm losing money every minute that we're closed.'

'How long do they think it's going to take?'

Cash shrugged. 'No one seems to be able to give me a definitive answer. But better now than when the season starts, I suppose. They put a little camera down the pipe earlier and seem to think they've found the problem. It's just a question of putting it right now. Anyway, enough about my drains. I can offer you a drink if you'd like one. It'd be good to catch up – but I can't even rustle something up for you in the kitchen because they've turned the bloody water off, unless you fancy a sandwich.'

Alex glanced at me. 'Nice offer, but we were hoping to sample the fish.'

'I'm really sorry. Would you like a glass of something, maybe? We've got a great cellar.' He tipped his head in invitation, while at the same time surreptitiously giving me the once over.

Clearly Alex hadn't told Cash that he was meeting anyone, but it seemed Alex wasn't going to give anything away. Instead he just sighed. 'I'm afraid not Cash. We're both driving so we can't even take you up on the wine. And there was me telling Sarah how wonderful the food is here.' He was teasing, laying on the disappointment with a trowel.

'That's right, he was,' I said, playing along.

Cash pulled a face. 'I'm so sorry. Another time. Next time the two of you are down this way come down and eat on the house. My treat.'

'I'm going to hold you to that. I was trying to impress Sarah with my good taste and great connections.'

'So are you two an item then?' asked Cash.

I laughed.

'What?' Cash protested. 'I'm always the last to know anything. Alex and I have been friends for years and he never tells me anything, so with him you don't know if you don't ask.'

Although Cash hadn't done it intentionally, that struck a nerve; one of the big problems with the relationship I had with Max was that he kept everything close to his chest and kept different aspects of his life in separate compartments. The problems had started when the walls between them had started to crumble – and I wasn't sure if I was ready to go through that with someone else.

I had to remind myself that comparisons are never a good thing. Even without knowing that much about Alex, I could already tell that he and Max were like chalk and cheese.

Max was always very formal, old school, with a refined, restrained manner in public and in private, whereas Alex seemed relaxed and – I hunted around for the right words to describe how he seemed; the best I could come up with was that he seemed emotionally available and generous, rather than closed off.

While I was thinking, Cash was asking how long we'd known each other.

Alex looked heavenwards. 'Excuse my friend,' he said. 'He always was nosey. If you must know, Cash, this is our first date and I brought Sarah here to impress her.'

'So, failed at the first hurdle then,' said Cash philosophically. 'Don't judge him too harshly, Sarah. He's not so bad once you get to know him. Although I could tell you a few stories about when we were at –'

'Well, don't,' said Alex, holding up a hand to silence him. 'I'd like to think we can have more than one date. Anyway, I don't know about Sarah but I'm absolutely famished, so as we're not going to be eating here can you suggest somewhere else local where we can go?' Alex asked.

Cash sighed. 'You want me to recommend the opposition?'

Alex nodded. 'Preferably open and not too far away.'

Cash now looked heavenwards. 'Okay ...'

Which was how we ended up sitting in a tiny little café on the seafront, less than a mile from Cash's place, eating fish and chips out of the paper. The place itself looked as if it hadn't changed much since the 1960s, but it was right on the promenade, was really busy and had the most fabulous view out over the sea, where that day the sky was so bright and so blue that it made my eyes water. Through the open door we could hear the gulls calling and squabbling as they spiralled above the incoming tide, while a flotilla of little boats bobbed at anchor in the tiny harbour.

The only place to eat inside the café was a high Formica-covered shelf that ran around the walls, which was about eighteen inches wide, dotted with glass salt and vinegar shakers and had bar stools tucked under it. Though the décor was very basic, nothing could detract from just how good the fish and chips were.

'Your friend was right. This is amazing,' I said, breaking off some more of the milky white fish flakes with my fingers and popping them into my mouth. 'I can't remember the last time I had fish and chips. It's really delicious.'

Alex grinned. 'It's not exactly what I had in mind. I was planning to woo you with my sophisticated charms and fine dining. Not fish and chips and a can of Fanta.'

I liked his easy charm and the way he wasn't fazed by the change of events and venue.

I smiled. 'Don't worry. I'm really enjoying this.'

'Me too,' he said, guiding a chip into his mouth. 'It's really tasty.'

So far, despite the shaky start, it was going really well. Better than well. It might not have been posh nosh, but we were having a great time. Alex was good company: funny, quick, and he seemed easy-going. He had spent a lot of his life travelling for his job and had loads of stories to tell, which he managed to do without sounding as if he was bragging or showing off. He made me laugh and he was happy to listen – and I knew he really was listening by the things he asked me. So far, so good. Alex had quiet self-assurance that was attractive and nice eyes that were hard to ignore.

I've got lots of rules about internet dating, one of them being to have a safe call in place so that a friend knows where I am and that I'm okay – in my case it was a text from a friend. If I am okay, I text back a pre-arranged reply. Anything else, including no reply, and she calls out the cavalry. The pre-arranged text is also a painless way to cut a bad date short. It goes like this: the text comes in, I peer at the screen, pull an anxious face, make my excuses and leave. With Alex my text from Gabbie had come and gone and we were still talking.

We had told each other about our jobs and families and gone through all the niceties that need to be gone through, before moving on to what had really brought us together for lunch. It was just a question of who broached the subject first.

'Have you been on many of these kinds of things?' Alex asked, dipping a chip into a little pot of sauce.

'You mean internet dates or trips to the chip shop?'

He laughed. 'Let's go with the dating first, shall we?'

'A few. Some straight and some –' I glanced over my shoulder at the other customers who were sitting no more than a couple of feet away from us, busily tucking into their own food. This was really not the place to go into the finer points of BDSM dating.

'Not so straight,' Alex suggested with a grin, catching my eye and, I suspect, my discomfort.

'Exactly, and it's been fun. I've met some really great people and some interesting ones and –'

'And ones that developed into a relationship?'

I nodded. 'Yes. Just the one.'

'So far,' Alex added with a smile.

'Yes, so far,' I conceded. 'My last relationship, his name was Max and I met him online on the same site where you found my profile.'

'And is this the one that was complicated?'

I nodded. 'I'm glad you were listening. Yes, it was complicated, but it was also wonderful – really good. I wouldn't have missed it for the world.'

'But it ended?'

'I ended it,' I said, and turned my attention back to my lunch.

I could see Alex watching my face, a clear invitation that he wanted to hear more, but I wasn't ready to tell him about Max and most certainly not in a crowded chip shop at the seaside.

'Long story,' I said, after a moment or two's silence. 'It's probably best saved for another time. How about you?' I asked.

'I've met a few women from the site we met on.' He looked round at the two plump elderly women sitting behind me, both cheerfully devouring their cod and chips and apparently oblivious to our conversation. 'Although I have done some online dating before. Tell you what,' he said. 'How do you fancy going for a walk once we've finished these? It might be easier to talk?'

Clearly he was right, but I hesitated before agreeing. Among my rules about internet dating is not putting myself in a situation where I'm alone with my date or away from other people.

I glanced out of the café window. Although it was late spring and the wind was fresh as it whipped in from the sea, there were quite a few people about, all well wrapped up against the cold, some of them walking dogs, some watching the boats bobbing about in the harbour, some just out for a stroll. Busy enough to be safe, I decided.

'Okay,' I said.

This meeting with Alex was very different from my first meeting with Max. When Max and I had met he had sent me a set of very precise instructions about how he wanted me to dress on our first date, and all kinds of formal terms and conditions about the nature of our relationship. When I'd asked Alex about what he wanted me to wear he'd said, 'Wear anything you want; I just want to meet you and get to know you. See how we get along. For me, it's about who you are, not whether you've got a mini-skirt and high heels on – although I like both of those things.'

So I'd taken Alex at his word and worn trousers and boots, which would have been a total no-no for Max, whose rules included my body being totally available to him whenever he wanted – so no bra, no knickers and stockings and suspenders or thigh-highs had been my standard subbie uniform, even in public, for all the time we were together, certainly not skinny jeans and boots.

For Max, who I was was important too, but the fact that I was prepared – from the very start – to do as he told me was also very important. Like I said, chalk and cheese.

I also realised that I had quite liked the rules and formality of Max's approach as a Dom. It had been great training for someone with no experience of submission, and I wondered how I would deal with someone new who seemed to have a much more relaxed approach. When we had finished eating Alex gathered up the debris from our lunch, dropped it in the bin and then offered me his arm.

'So,' he said, as we set off along the promenade, 'are you going to tell me about Max?'

'You first,' I said.

'What do you want to know about me?'

'Everything,' I said.

'Okay, but you realise I'm expecting this to be reciprocal?'

I nodded.

'Okay. Do you fancy an ice cream?' he said, as we passed a brightly painted booth. 'How about we have a ninety-nine?'

I laughed. An ice-cream cone with a chocolate flake in it was hardly part of the lunch with a sophisticated Dom-about-town that I had envisaged. 'Come on,' Alex said, taking my hand and guiding me over to the window. 'It's been years since I've had one.' He glanced into the kiosk. 'Oh my God, look, they've got sprinkles!' he said, turning round and grinning at me.

How I could I possibly resist?

'So,' he said, as we walked away with a huge ice cream each, complete with flakes and enough hundreds and thousands to sink a battleship. 'BDSM. I was probably in my mid-twenties when I started to fantasise about tying women up and doing all sorts of weird and wonderful things to them while they were helpless. I'd had the thoughts before, but that was when I first realised that I wanted to turn it into a reality.' Before he went into any more detail Alex glanced at me as if to gauge my reaction.

I'd been there. I knew how hard it was to voice those secret desires that don't just excite you, but also make you feel ashamed of what you're thinking and feeling and wanting, and make you anxious about the way your mind works. We all have different values and ideas about sexual behaviour, but I think most of us would concede that what practice. It wasn't like I wanted to torture anyone though,' he said quickly, and then he grinned when he saw that I hadn't flinched or run away screaming. 'Okay, well, maybe torture them just a little bit, maybe nipple clamps and some other toys and a riding crop, things like that, but no real pain. For me, it's not so much about inflicting pain as about having the power of being in control, of being able to take my time and set the agenda, of having someone surrender totally to me. Anyway, despite it figuring in a lot of my fantasies, I also came to the conclusion that I probably shouldn't mention it to anyone in case I got arrested.'

I couldn't help but laugh. Alex was right; suggest this and most women would run a mile, but I'm not most women, nor am I alone in what I feel or how I enjoy my sexual encounters. I genuinely love and enjoy what Alex was describing as long as what is done is consensual and shared with someone I like and respect and above all feel safe with and trust. Alex, meanwhile, was still speaking.

'Four years ago I split up with Lucy and I met a woman on a vanilla dating site who was into bondage. I didn't know that when we first met. In fact, I'm not even sure now how we got onto the subject – I think maybe we'd both had a glass or two of wine and both of us had been itching to try it and to find someone who wasn't shocked. Anyway, we *did* talk about it and after that we played a little bit. She liked me to tie her to the bed, and that was about all, to be honest, but from the very first moment I realised just how much it excited me. It felt so right. We talked a lot and went looking at all sorts of websites together. The biggest relief and realisation was that I wasn't alone in liking that kind of thing and that there were women out there, like her and you, who wanted to play too. It was something I knew I wanted to explore further.'

'So what happened?'

'I hadn't long split up with my wife and at that point neither of us were looking for anything serious. We saw each other for a few months but gradually drifted apart. And then I dated on and off, went on some vanilla sites and very gently broached it with other women. Some were keen, some weren't – and I slowly realised that actually it was something I wanted to be able to share and talk openly about with my partner, not pussyfoot around, worried that they'd call the police or run a mile.'

'Which is why we're here,' I said.

He nodded.

'So you were on the site for quite a while?'

'Yes, although you were the first person I ever rang on the BDSM website. I emailed a couple of others and, as you were taken,' he said with a grin, 'I met a few of them, but they weren't right and frankly I'd rather be on my own than in the wrong relationship.'

'Me too. So have you been on your own since we last spoke?'

'On and off. I've had a few dates, but nothing that was going anywhere.'

'And is that what you're looking for? Something that is going somewhere?'

Alex nodded. 'In an ideal world, but I'm in no hurry, so –' he smiled, 'no pressure.'

Being with someone new and possibly even greener than me wasn't something I had factored into my search for a Dom. I'd liked Max initially because it felt like he knew what he was doing. As if reading my mind, Alex said: 'I've just never been with someone who I've known is submissive right from the start.'

I raised my eyebrows. 'You do understand that being a submissive doesn't mean that I'm either stupid or a doormat, don't you?'

'I never assumed that for a moment,' he said, holding his hands – and ice cream – up.

'Good,' I said. 'Most of the subs I've met are really strong women. They're just looking for a stronger man, someone who can understand them. Someone who can handle them.'

'In both senses of the word?'

'In an ideal world,' I said, echoing his comment of a few moments earlier.

It was tricky talking hard-core sex with a man who had a sprinkle of hundreds and thousands on his nose. I reached out to wipe them off and he smiled as I touched him.

'I'm really glad you decided to come today,' he said. 'I was disappointed when I rang before and you said you'd met someone. I felt like I'd been cheated out of something special.'

It was an odd thing to say; not creepy or stalker-like, just unsettling. And there was a moment then when we were so close that I thought Alex might kiss me – which was also odd because in BDSM, despite the intimate relationship between a Dom and their sub, often they don't kiss. Max had told me that kissing was for lovers, not Masters and their sex slaves. But I realised as Alex and I moved apart and the moment passed that I had wanted him to kiss me.

'It's a real shame we don't know each other better,' Alex said, taking my arm as he helped me down over the harbour wall. 'I'm going to a wedding in Whitby at the end of next week. Old family friends. I was going to make it a three-day trip. You could have come with me. I've booked into a really nice hotel.'

I looked at him and laughed. Outrageous! 'You think I'm going to be swayed by the promise of a couple of nights in a half-decent hotel?'

'You never know your luck,' Alex said with a shrug.

'You're really not backwards in coming forwards, are you?'

Alex smiled, eyes bright with mischief. 'It's not something I've ever been accused of, no. How about you? How forward are you?' he teased.

'I'm not,' I said primly, realising that I sounded more like a schoolmistress than a submissive.

'Okay, not a problem,' he said. 'Maybe next time. The friend whose daughter is getting married has got six kids. I'm sure this won't be the last time I get an invite to see one of them get married. And it's a lovely part of the world. Have you ever been?'

I shook my head.

'Amazing countryside, and Whitby is a real little gem.'

By now we had wandered way down past the boats and onto the beach where only the hardiest were walking in the cutting wind. I glanced across at Alex, wrapped up in a Barbour jacket, scarf tucked in, his head down, and smiled. He was lovely and, mad as this may sound, that set every alarm bell in my head ringing. What exactly was I thinking? Lovely? Hadn't I said I'd take my time, not get involved, treat this as a trial run? *Lovely?* It was total madness.

What were the chances of walking out of one relationship straight into another one that was right? Next to zero, I'd have said. If I had drawn up a wish list of what I wanted in a man I suspect Alex would have ticked practically every box, and that was my dilemma. I didn't believe what I was feeling and I didn't trust myself or my instincts. Maybe it was because I hadn't been out with anyone for so long.

The problem I was having was that the chemistry thing, which is usually so elusive and so very hard to find with someone, was there, so tangible that you'd have to have been dead not to feel it. I fancied Alex, and I knew damn well that he fancied me, and the fact was it terrified me.

What if this was a rebound thing or just lust? Was it that Max had created a need in me – like a drug habit – that longed to be fed? There was a good chance that this man could fulfil that need; was that what made me think I fancied him? I didn't trust my instincts. Alex was lovely and there was a part of me – the mad, reckless part – that thought actually a few days in Whitby with him sounded like huge fun. But that wasn't what I said. Instead I stuffed my hands into the pockets of my jacket and tucked my head down to avoid the cutting wind and said nothing.

'I'll book you into a separate room,' Alex said. 'No strings. Or ropes, or anything even vaguely bondage. How does that sound?'

I laughed. 'Boring.'

He threw back his head and laughed along with me. While I believed Alex when he said that he would book separate rooms, I think both of us knew that if I went to Whitby with him that wasn't what was going to happen.

# Chapter Three

'For God's sake,' said Gabbie, pouring me another glass of wine. 'You're hardly a blushing virgin. Go. It'll do you good.'

'You make it sound like some sort of universal cure-all.'

'Nothing wrong with a little therapeutic sex, Sarah. Come on, you said yourself that he is cute, and let's face it, you could do with a diversion. You've been moping about for months since you split up with Max. Time to start over, honey. Time to be getting on with life.'

'I have been getting on with life,' I protested.

She raised her eyebrows. 'As far as I can see you've been getting on with avoiding life,' she said.

Gabbie is one of my best and oldest friends. Along with Joan and Helen, we make up a quartet of friends who go back the best part of twenty-five years, and we are still going strong. The four of us first met up at antenatal classes in a draughty scout hut on the outskirts of Cambridge, but we've all come an awfully long way since then. When our children were small we used to meet up once a month at each other's houses. Now that we've all moved away and moved on and our children have grown up, we still try to get together regularly for supper, it just doesn't happen as often as any of us would like.

Tonight, however, was an extraordinary mid-week general meeting with just Gabbie and me present, because I thought Joan would disapprove of me going away with Alex on principle and Helen had started seeing a man called Geoff and was so excited and loved up that – pleased as I was – I knew that he would be the main topic of conversation. Even if we did talk about Alex and the pros and cons of going away with a complete stranger for a dirty weekend, she wouldn't really be listening and, while I didn't want to steal her thunder, I needed some support and advice. Helen deserved a good man. We all did.

'I don't know why you're making such a big thing of this. What harm can it do?' Gabbie was saying. We had ordered a takeaway. She was waving an onion bhaji around for added emphasis. 'You're a big girl now, Sarah. You don't need anyone's approval, least of all mine. Look at the mess I make of relationships. Go to Whitby, have a good time, have a weekend in a nice hotel with someone you fancy and have some good meaningless sex. Or not. Let him book you a separate room and have a bit of a cuddle. Your choice. You're old enough to make up your own mind now, and you can have a relationship any shape you want it to be these days. I mean, he might be *the one*.'

I laughed. 'Yes, and he could also be an axe murderer.'

'True. But then again so could anyone else you go out with and –'

'He offered to drive,' I said.

'And what? Your mother was very strict about you getting into cars with strangers?'

'And rightly so.'

'Okay, so you offer to drive up there then.'

'I don't want to drive to Whitby. It's bloody miles away.'

'Go by train and meet him there.'

'It'll take all day.'

'Okay, well, don't go at all then,' said Gabbie, throwing up her hands in frustration.

'But I want to go,' I said, realising that with every passing minute I was sounding more and more like a petulant teenager than a fortysomething adult with a job, a mortgage and grown-up kids.

'You probably know a lot more about Alex than you would about some guy you'd met in a bar, and I think you'd know if he was weird.'

'You'd like to think so, wouldn't you? But I'm not sure I trust my instincts.'

'Oh well, that's it then. Ring him up and tell him you're not going. Or do you want me to do it?' Gabbie paused and waited for me to reply, and when I didn't she said, 'What you really want is for me to give you my approval and to encourage you to go, don't you?'

She was right, of course. I just needed someone else to tell me it was okay and I wasn't mad to want to go away with him.

To help convince me that he wasn't weird or a mad man, Alex had sent me a map of where we would be staying, a link to the hotel website, a copy of the wedding invitation and all sorts of numbers and bits and bobs so that I could check him and his invitation out. If he was an axe murderer he had gone to an awful lot of trouble to make himself look credible.

When we'd parted in the car park after our day out at the seaside, he had kissed me very briefly and told me to let him know if I wanted to go with him to the wedding. He said it would be great to spend some more time together, and part of me agreed wholeheartedly. The afternoon had just flown by and I hadn't had such a nice time in ages. He had such a light touch on life, and had made me laugh more in one afternoon than I had in weeks. He had made me smile and he had listened, and made me realise that there was life after Max, and that without meaning to I had been wallowing in a whole world of 'poor me', even if I hadn't said anything out loud.

'So,' Alex had said as we got to my car. 'Time to go then.'

I nodded as he bobbed in to kiss me on the cheek. 'I've had a great time,' he said.

'Me too,' I said. I didn't want him to go and it seemed the feeling was mutual because he ran through the plan for Whitby one more time.

Alex planned to drive up on Thursday morning, then go to the wedding on Friday and come back on Saturday. Or Sunday, he offered, still smiling. As he spoke, I wondered if he might kiss me for real, rather than the maiden-aunt-style peck he'd just given me. At which point he leant in closer, and I felt my heart do that fluttery thing that hearts do – and I almost pulled away, coming over all prudish, as I felt a surge of what felt remarkably like pure old-fashioned lust. And then he kissed me properly and I was convinced of it. It was lust, pure and simple, and it was heady stuff. I'd been through a lean time. His kiss was like nectar.

I can't remember the last time that kissing someone genuinely made me go weak at the knees, but Alex's kiss came damned close. Good kissing is an art – this was close to perfect; he gently held me by the elbows, bringing me into range, and then he brushed my lips with his. The kiss was just intimate enough; strong but not too pushy, gentle pressure and slightly open mouth but no tongues, with the promise of more to come. When he pulled away, Alex's eyes were bright with a flicker of desire and a lot of amusement. He grinned. 'I'd really like to do a lot more of that. Have a safe trip home.'

I felt myself blushing and then he was gone.

By the time I got back to my place Alex had already texted me: 'Great to spend time with you today. I've emailed you the details of the wedding, but seriously, no pressure. I'd really love to see you again, whether you come to the wedding or not. Just hoping you feel the same. A x'

Across my kitchen table, between plates and takeaway cartons, Gabbie turned my laptop round to face her. 'We could always ring the venue and make sure the wedding is for real.'

I stared at her. 'You think he would *fake* a wedding?'

'I don't know, do I? I wasn't the one who met him.'

'I'm sure he wouldn't. He was really nice, good company, tall, blond, broad shoulders, and I really fancied him,' I said, scooping up the last of the saag with a piece of naan bread.

'So what's your problem?' said Gabbie.

'What if I'm wrong?'

Gabbie stared at me. 'About what? Him being nice or faking a wedding?'

'Fancying him.'

'Are you planning to marry him?'

I stared at her. 'No, of course not. I've only just met him.'

'Right, well, in that case lighten up for God's sake. Just go and see how you get on. You're over-thinking this, Sarah.' Gabbie pulled out her mobile from her handbag and reading from the screen tapped in a number.

'What on earth are you doing?' I asked.

'Ringing the hotel so we can check up on Mr Tall-Blond-with-Broad-Shoulders,' Gabbie said. Then, before I could protest, she continued in a warm, super-cheery voice: 'Oh, hello there, I'm just ringing to check up on a booking we made for later this week. Mr Alex Fallon?' She paused for a moment or two, listening to whoever was at the other end, and then continued, 'That's right. Coming up for a wedding. Yes, that's it, booked in on – yes – that's great. I just wanted to make sure he's got it all sorted. You know what men are like. Thursday for two nights? That's great, thank you so much, that's lovely,' she gushed, and with that Gabbie hung up.

'Are they allowed to do that?' I asked in amazement.

'You just have to get the voice right, and there you go – so far his story adds up. Double room, single occupancy for two nights is what the lady said, but then again I suppose anyone can book a hotel, although booking it a fortnight ago shows some forward planning if he is making it all up.' I knew Gabbie was teasing me, but it wasn't helping. She turned her attention back to the screen and started to tap another number into the phone.

'What the hell are you doing now?'

'I was going to call the RSVP number,' Gabbie said mischievously. 'Get it straight from the horse's mouth.'

'Don't you dare,' I said, trying to snatch the phone out of her hand.

'I'm only joking, but maybe we ought to ring the wedding venue and check that out too?'

One thing I should say is that Gabbie doesn't know that I'm into BDSM – as far as she is concerned Max was just another man, and Alex too. I'm not sure what she would think of the BDSM thing and, much as I love her, I've never told her. I'm worried that she won't understand.

Gabbie, meanwhile, was back on the phone. 'Hello?' she said. 'I'm just ringing to make sure I've got the right place. We're coming up for a wedding this Friday and I wanted to make sure that we end up at the right one.' She laughed; someone at the other end of the line laughed too. 'The name of the wedding party? Certainly.' Gabbie read the names of the bride and groom off the screen and nodded in response to whoever she was speaking to. 'That's lovely – no, we're really looking forward to it. Oh right, that's great. I'll take a look on your website. Fine. See you soon. And thank you – that's really helpful.'

Gabbie glanced across at me. 'So far, so good. She said all I needed to do was put the postcode into my sat nav. Apparently they're very easy to find and they're really looking forward to seeing me. So, little Miss Prim-and-Proper, have you made up your mind?'

I glanced at my plate. 'What the hell do you wear to the wedding of people you don't know?'

Gabbie handed me her phone. 'Why don't you ring Alex and find out?' she said, spooning the last of the rogan josh onto her plate.

Which was why the following Thursday I found myself sitting in the passenger seat of Alex's TT, heading up the coast road towards Whitby with a hatbox balanced on my knees and a genuine sense of excitement and anticipation. We'd stopped for lunch in York and then taken a detour off the main route so we could see the sea. It was a good choice.

It was the most perfect early-spring day and you could see for miles. The other good news was that on a second viewing Alex was just as fanciable and just as good company as he had been the first time around, and we were getting on like a house on fire. We'd talked about family and friends and holidays and places we had been and places we'd still like to go. The drive was pretty much uneventful except for Alex announcing one slight change of plan.

Since we had spoken on the phone he had swapped hotels and hotel rooms with one of the bride's family because the room Alex had been booked into was on the ground floor, and the family member had small children and was worried that the wedding-venue hotel, full of celebrating newlyweds and their guests, would be too noisy. So we now had a suite at the wedding venue with two adjoining rooms. Alex insisted that I let Gabbie know where I was, just in case she (or I) was worried and felt the need to check up on me. As I got into the car he had handed me a sheet of paper with the new number and details on it and insisted that I text her.

We had talked for hours about our lives and our families, but as we drove down the hill towards the coast and our destination, Alex, whose eyes were firmly fixed on the road, said, 'We haven't talked much about the main reason we're both here.'

I glanced across at him.

'Don't worry. I'm just glad that you said you'd come. I understand if you don't want to play for whatever reason, or if you want to wait until we know each other better. If you don't want to play, then we'll just have a great weekend away and call it quits. There is no pressure whatsoever, but if you do want to play you'll have to ask me.'

'Ask you?'

Alex nodded. 'If you want to play.'

I felt a little ripple of excitement and smiled. It seemed to me Doms were big on making you ask for what you wanted; maybe they got a kick out of hearing a woman beg. 'What do you want me to say?'

He grinned. 'I don't mind. Anything you want.'

I hesitated. Wasn't this what I wanted? Wasn't this why I was here? With Max, before he and I had got to this stage we had exchanged lots of emails about what he expected from his submissive, and before there had been any physical contact we'd both signed a contract, which outlined the rules of engagement and included safe words, what he and I would commit to and the boundaries we had both agreed on.

'What about safe words and limits?' I asked Alex.

'We can sort that out as we go. I want us both to be able to explore this – although if you want a contract then I'm sure we can draw one up, but before we get to that point I need you to ask me.'

I stared at him and unexpectedly felt my eyes filling up with tears. I wasn't sure that I was ready for this. I wanted to play, but maybe it was too early for me to start over. I barely knew Alex and I wondered if he really knew what being a Dom meant.

Alex glanced across at me. 'Are you okay?' he said, and when he realised that maybe I wasn't, he pulled the car over to the side of the road. 'I'm sorry, I didn't mean to upset you.'

I laughed and wiped away the tears. 'You haven't, I'm *so* sorry. I'm absolutely fine. I don't know where that came from. It's just me being stupid. I got myself emotionally mashed first time round when I did this. And yes, I do want to play, but we might need to take it slowly.'

He handed me a tissue. 'That's okay. But you still have to ask me.'

I nodded.

'And while we're together and while we play you will call me Sir from now on, although if, after this weekend, or even during this weekend, you feel as if you've made a mistake or it's too much then that's okay – no hard feelings, we can just cool it down or walk away. Okay?'

I nodded. I understood. It was what I wanted and needed too. 'Yes, Sir,' I said.

He smiled. 'Now, ask me,' he said.

Ds (Dom-sub) relationships are no less passionate or emotionally intense than any other kind of relationship between two people, but there is usually, in my experience, far more negotiation, more discussion, before there is any sexual contact, which to those outside listening in can make it sound more like a transaction than attraction.

Most of the Ds couples and singles I've talked to over the years don't, as a rule, however fast they move from fancying to getting physical, just fall into bed with each other after a first drunken night out and have crazy drunken Ds sex. I'm not saying it doesn't happen, just not with the people I've talked to. For one thing, it's way too dangerous to play hard when you're drunk.

By the time a Dom and sub get to the point where they want to play with each other – play being the term used to describe a Ds scenario – they've talked about what they want, what they like and what they don't like, which, let's face it, isn't the way most vanilla relationships go. From the outside it may sound colder, but in fact it's fun; it builds trust, confidence and connections. Even if you are wildly attracted, in my experience the encounters – at least at the outset – are much more structured until you know your way around each other and what you like and don't like.

Lust, desire, love, passion: they are all there, but the way Ds couples negotiate their way through the beginning of their relationships is just a little different from what most people are used to.

So, I was agreeing that, for this weekend, maybe longer, Alex would be my dominant man, a Dom, *my* Dom – the man who, when we were playing, could tell me what to do. By my acknowledging him in that role I was giving him permission to use and explore my body as he saw fit within the boundaries we had agreed. As his sub I would choose to submit to him. In many ways I would give myself to him. It is heady and powerful stuff.

One thing I had learned early on from being with Max is that you can't give what you don't have. To be able to submit to someone you have to know who you are and be strong enough to let go.

So, sitting in the TT on the side of the coast road a long, long way from home, I said: 'Please, Sir. Can we play?'

Alex smiled at me and nodded. 'Yes, we can. I've been thinking about this since we met last weekend.' The amusement was back in his eyes. 'I've got such plans for you.'

# Chapter Four

Alex and I arrived at the hotel in the middle of the afternoon. It was in an old country house a few miles outside Whitby and was beyond fabulous. With the house set in a great stand of trees and tucked up among acres of rolling parkland, the hotel owners had managed to keep the feel of old-fashioned genteel splendour and faded glamour alongside twenty-first-century convenience.

The entrance hall was like something from a movie set – *The Great Gatsby* or maybe something by Agatha Christie – with great sofas and fireplaces, crystal chandeliers and ornate side tables, and the centrepiece being a grand staircase that swept up from a black-and-white tiled floor to Lord only knew where. The reception desk was set discreetly to one side and staffed by a bevy of smiling, efficient young women in uniform.

As Alex was booking us in a gaggle of wedding guests appeared from nowhere and practically mugged him with their sheer exuberance. It struck me that in some ways this was the perfect way to find out about anyone; there really is no hiding place at a family wedding, and any lingering concerns I might have had about Alex were rapidly snuffed out by the obvious delight the other wedding guests took in seeing him.

There were several couples, single girls and small children and a couple of elderly grannies. Alex made the introductions, though the names came and went; this one was a long-lost friend of the family, this one a cousin from Australia, this someone's best friend from childhood. It seemed that they were all heading into the sitting room for afternoon tea and they were very keen for us to join them.

Alex smiled at me. 'We'd love to but it's been a really long drive, and Sarah and I need to get unpacked and settled in.' He glanced at his watch. 'We've got a few things to do. We're probably going to be tied up for an hour or two – maybe we could meet up for dinner?'

The play on words wasn't lost on me, nor was the look Alex gave me.

As Alex said his farewells and made promises to meet up later, the porter took our bags and we headed up the impressive staircase into the main hotel.

'Aren't you taking a risk bringing someone you don't know to something like this?' I said, *sotto voce*. 'I mean, I could be a real liability – mad or a drinker or anything.'

'Are you?' he asked.

'Well, no, but –'

Alex laughed. 'I didn't think so, and anyway it was a risk I was prepared to take. I wanted to spend some real time with you.'

'Even if it meant me kicking off in front of the bride and groom?'

Alex laughed and took my arm. 'I think I can probably handle it.'

Beyond the vast lobby and the first-floor landing the hotel was a complete rabbit warren. Within moments of getting upstairs I was not only lost, but totally disorientated – all the busy sounds from the reception area were completely deadened by miles of flock wallpaper and deep-pile carpets and the hallways were long, silent and stately. The walls were hung with magnificent paintings, there were fabulous flower arrangements and statuary in niches all along the walls and antique furniture that looked as if it had been there forever.

'This way, sir, madam,' said our guide, as after what seemed like a long hike he finally opened the doors to our room. The suite was in one corner of the hotel in a turret, with mullioned windows that overlooked a carefully manicured knot garden. There was a Jack and Jill bathroom between the two large airy bedrooms. The main room had a huge four-poster bed and antique furniture, while the smaller room had a queen-sized bed and looked like a typical boutique hotel room with cushions and throws and contemporary art. Both rooms were stylish and luxurious enough to pull off the contrast.

As the man deposited our bags, Alex looked long and hard at the four-poster, and then at me, and raised his eyebrows in unspoken invitation as we both took in the very thing that had first sparked his fantasies. The porter left with a healthy tip.

'Let's start nice and slowly,' Alex said, as soon as the doors were closed and we were alone. 'Take off your clothes.'

'That counts as slowly, does it?' I said with amusement.

'Does it, *Sir*,' said Alex.

I laughed again; this was horribly familiar territory for me. I'm not good at remembering to call anyone Sir, and Max had taken great pleasure in punishing me every time I forgot.

'And while we're playing you will only speak when spoken to. Do you understand?' Alex asked.

Only too well. I nodded.

'Now, undress for me.'

Alex settled himself down into one of the leather armchairs in the bay window of the turret. His expression was fixed and neutral. He was waiting to see what I would do and I knew in some ways that this was the first test. The room was totally silent now except for the tick-tick-tick of a long-case clock that was standing against one wall. It seemed like time slowed as I lifted my fingers to the buttons of my jacket.

I am not by nature any kind of exhibitionist; the idea of undressing in front of someone I barely know comes with all kinds of fears and anxieties, and the added frisson of embarrassment and self-consciousness in many ways adds to the intensity of the moment. Submission is about embracing all those feelings and letting them feed your arousal. I was trembling, excited, anxious – awash with a whole raft of adrenaline-fuelled emotions as I let my jacket drop to the floor. Under the jacket I was wearing a fitted floral dress that buttoned all the way down the front. The buttons were tiny, and under Alex's penetrating gaze my fingers seemed too big, too clumsy to deal with them. One by one they gave way. I could feel him watching me, watching my progress, button by button, until finally the dress fell open.

As I slipped it back off my shoulders I heard the breath catch in his throat. I knew without a doubt that I had every molecule of his attention. I smiled inwardly; Max had been the first one to point out to me that in reality it was often the sub who wielded the most power. Alex was just as hooked on this moment as I was. Under my dress I was wearing a black lacy bra, matching knickers and stockings and suspenders, along with black court shoes. I let the dress drop to the floor.

'God, you are lovely,' Alex murmured, getting to his feet. I felt myself blush. 'Turn around for me. I want to look at you,' he continued.

I did as I was told. He walked around me as I turned, his eyes working their way hungrily over my body, inspecting me, taking in every inch of me. His gaze was as exciting and invasive as any caress. His attention, his obvious desire and pleasure were intoxicating.

'Very nice,' he said, in a voice barely above a whisper. 'Now take off your bra.'

I fumbled with the catch. Alex waited. As it gave way I slipped off the shoulder straps, instinctively holding the flimsy fabric in place in front of my body, a nod towards modesty.

'Here,' he said, holding out his hand towards me. 'I want to look at your breasts. I want to look at all of you.'

I dropped the bra into his open palm while I covered my breasts with my forearm.

'Put your hands on top of your head.' He spoke with a quiet assurance. This was an order, not a request. I did as he told me. My nipples hardened in the cool air. Alex smiled. 'Wonderful. You are exquisite. This is going to be so much fun, Sarah. I've been thinking about this moment since I met you. Come here.'

He beckoned me over. 'You are beautiful,' he murmured.

I am neither exquisite nor beautiful, but it seems to me that men are so much less critical than we women and see so much more in us than we do in ourselves. They see beauty and loveliness where we only see lumps and bumps and cellulite.

I stepped towards him and he cupped my breasts, his thumbs working back and forth across the hard, dark buds of my nipples. He bent down and took first one and then the other into his mouth, sucking gently. I closed my eyes, my body soaking up the sensations. I groaned softly. I heard him chuckle as he pulled away.

'Seems like I'm not the only one who needs this,' he said.

I opened my eyes. He was so close that I could see the stubble on the side of his face where he hadn't quite caught it with the razor and smell the soft scent of his body and hair. He made my mouth water.

'Are you okay?' He whispered, tipping my face up towards him.

I nodded.

'Tell me,' he said.

I smiled. 'I'm fine. Nervous, excited, but fine.'

'Good. Because I want you to enjoy every second of this. I'm going to beat you and then I am going to fuck you,' he said, in an undertone. 'And I need to know that that is what you want. Is that what you want, Sarah?'

I stared at him. 'We haven't got a safe word,' I began.

'"Whitby". If you want me to stop say "Whitby". Now tell me that you want me to beat you.'

Our eyes met. It was the moment when we both stepped from what might be considered acceptable into the realms of otherness that BDSM occupies. Before I had given him my answer Alex stepped away from me and unfastened one of the cases that the porter had set down on an ottoman at the end of the bed. He took out a riding crop.

I watched him, hypnotised, entranced, torn between how much I longed to feel the sensations and the rush of endorphins that I knew followed the bite of the crop as it hit home and knowing just how much being cropped hurt.

Alex flexed the plaited leather shaft, his eyes not leaving mine as he did it. The crop was new, unyielding. I swallowed hard.

'I need you to tell me that this is what you want, Sarah, or we don't go any further. And if that is the case, it's fine, but I need to know. What do you want?'

I had been here before with Max. My throat was dry, the words wouldn't come.

Alex waited. 'Well?' he said quietly. 'What do you say?'

'Yes, please,' I murmured, ever polite.

He smiled. 'Good. Get hold of the arms of the chair and bend over.'

I stepped towards the chair, taking a deep breath, preparing myself for what was to come.

'Wait,' he said. 'Take off your knickers.'

With my back to him, I slipped them down over my hips and let them fall to the floor, imagining the view of my lily-white bum framed by black suspenders and the tops of my stockings.

'Very nice,' Alex purred, as he ran a hand appreciatively over the curve of my backside and then, with his palm on the small of my back, guided me down over the leather armchair. The only way to do it and be comfortable was to open my legs.

As I did Alex's hand slipped down over my tailbone, down lower, caressing all my most intimate places, working towards the delicate folds of my sex, his nimble fingers exploring, dipping into me. Alex didn't need to tell me that I was wet. He made a little sound of pleasure as he took the time to explore my compliant, hungry body. I shivered as his fingers opened me, stroking and teasing. I pressed back onto him, pushing his fingers deeper.

'Bad girl, bad girl,' he said, stepping away from me. 'You know how this works. You have to wait until later, until you've earned it. First the pain and then the pleasure.'

I guessed what was coming next. I closed my eyes and waited, trying hard not to tense up, which I knew would only make the pain more intense.

Alex's first stroke with the crop was tentative, almost gentle, barely more than a tap. It made me wonder if he had ever cropped someone before, but actually I was glad that the blow was so gentle. It had been so long since I had played with anyone. After all the anticipation I'd been feeling over the last few days I wanted to relish it. I certainly didn't want to shriek and frighten Alex off or use the safe word if I could possibly help it. The second stroke was a little harder, but not much.

'We'll take this slowly,' he said, almost as if he could read my thoughts. There was the slightest tremor in his voice. I wasn't sure if it was nerves or excitement. 'We'll build it up gradually, a little at a time. I've brought a whole bag full of toys with me,' said Alex. 'Next time you can choose.'

I laughed and he hit me again, a little harder this time.

'Count,' he said.

'Three,' I said.

'Well done,' he said, and hit me again.

'Four.' This one was lower down, catching the top of my thighs. It stung like crazy and made me gasp, and as I gasped the crop found its mark again.

I stamped my feet, an involuntary reaction to the pain, as my hands flew round to rub the back of my thighs and the weal that rose within seconds. 'Five,' I said, through gritted teeth.

Alex teased the end of the crop backwards and forwards over my fingertips, guiding them away. 'Put your hands back on the arms of the chair and stay still,' ordered Alex. 'Now.'

It is very hard to just let someone hit you with a crop. Very hard to obey when you know that it will hurt. And sometimes the sensations create something like a tidal wave, a sensory overload, so it's hard to back down from them and tolerate any more. The stinging snap across my thighs was one of those sensations. I was trembling, suffused by a rolling heat and pain.

'Now,' he repeated more crisply.

I was close to that place. I slowly put my hands back, taking a deep breath, letting the tension ease away. Crazy as it might sound, I wanted this. I needed it. The last thing I wanted was to call a halt. I took another deep breath.

The next blow was squarely across my bum and though it made me gasp it was more bearable.

'How many is that?' Alex said.

'Six,' I hissed. I had forgotten that I was meant to count.

'Good girl.' The next blow made me cry out and realise how naïve I had been thinking the first few strokes had been too soft or that Alex didn't know what he was doing. He knew. He knew very, very well.

'Seven.'

I sucked in a ragged breath. My pulse was racing. I felt as if I was drowning in the rush of sensations as Alex hit me again.

'Eight.'

As the pain rippled through me I realised that I had forgotten just how much I love and hate this feeling. I swallowed hard. I had missed this so much and yet I was struggling with just how intense, how overwhelming it felt.

'Nine.' And I am consumed by the sensations, falling, falling into the void, my voice sounds a long, long way off; the pain is not.

'Ten.' I wonder fleetingly if Alex will stop at ten as I close my eyes tightly. Behind my closed eyes I can see the pain roaring through me like a coloured flare.

'Eleven.'

I have my answer.

'Twelve.'

And then there's a moment's stillness. Alex drops the crop onto the floor alongside the chair, takes my hands and leads me over to the bed. Eyes dark with desire he lifts me up and sets me down on the huge four-poster, in among the cushions and bolsters. He is breathing fast and heavy. I can sense his excitement, matching my own, as he kisses my neck, my throat, my breasts, my belly.

I moan with pure pleasure. Without pulling away he starts to unbutton his shirt and, desperate not to lose the moment, I am with him, undressing him too. We are both so hungry for this. His body is strong and muscular, the muscles clearly defined; his chest is broad and hairy, every inch a man. His hands work on his belt, freeing his cock, erect and full. He is beautiful. I reach out to touch him but he hasn't done with me yet.

Alex's hands explore every last inch of me, and where his fingers lead his tongue follows. As his tongue works lower and lower, moving down, down over my breasts and belly I am completely lost, lifting myself up towards him, eager and brazen. As his tongue finds the hard, throbbing bud of my clitoris I cry out in delight, demanding more as he licks and laps and sucks, his hands under my buttocks lifting me onto his tongue. God, he is good. I'm sobbing with pure ecstasy.

I can feel the storm building, feel the pleasure arcing, feel myself about to tumble over the edge, and then Alex is pulling away and I am begging for him to finish what he started – not leave me hanging – and then I realise that he is putting on a condom and as I reach out towards him, he eases himself slowly into me. I feel my body opening under him, feel his beautiful cock slide slowly deeper and deeper.

Buried to the hilt, he fills me to the brim. I fit tight around him and he starts to move, oh so slowly, with magnificent control, angling his pelvis so that he brushes up against the rise of my sex, brushing my clitoris with every stroke, the lightest touch of his skin against mine. I can't believe how good it feels. It is amazing, all-engulfing. I hold my breath as he moves again and then finally, blissfully let go, relishing the feelings as he oh-so-slowly fucks me.

I suspect that Alex won't be able to hang on for much longer; his breath is ragged and shallow, and I am as close to the edge as he is. He pushes deeper, I move with him, and I feel my body responding, arching up to meet his. And then, just as I feel the first white-hot ripples of orgasm, Alex looks into my eyes. His are dark with hunger and need and things that have no words, only feelings, and I am falling over the edge into the void. As I begin to come, I feel the first mesmerising pulse of his orgasm deep inside me, feel my sex close tight around him, feel the heat and the waves rolling through us both, making my body arch and stiffen under his, driving on and on until finally we are both totally spent and we collapse, breathing hard, falling down onto the bed, all passion expended, all tension gone.

Alex slides out of me and after a moment or two we curl up together, my back to his belly, his arms tight around me. I shiver with a mixture of cold and the remnants of excitement. In response he drags the corner of the bedcover up over both of us, and within seconds I am asleep in his arms, totally exhausted, utterly drained and blissfully content.

'So,' said Lisa, that night over dinner, 'how did you two meet?' She was looking at Alex, but the question was aimed fair and square at me. Lisa was the bride's youngest sister. She was slim, dark haired, dressed to kill, and was somewhere in her late teens or early twenties. According to the rest of the diners at our table, Lisa was the noisiest and nosiest of the family's six children. It was a close-run thing though; they were all noisy and funny, and full of stories and nonsense. Everyone, including me, was having a great time.

'Lisa, will you just stop it,' said Cathie, the bride's mother, in mock exasperation. All of the girls bore a strik-ing resemblance to her, and I'd liked Cathie as soon as we were introduced. Sitting alongside her, the bride, Carol, rolled her eyes.

'You can't take her anywhere. It's none of your business, nosey,' Cathie chided.

The wedding party had taken over most of the hotel and we had been invited to join what turned out to be a table of twelve, made up of the family of the bride, who was presently sitting between Cathie, her mum and her aunty. Carol was all beautifully spray-tanned, eyebrows plucked, looking sparkly, fresh and gorgeous, all ready for the big day.

In the bar, when Alex had tried to buy them a drink, the girls had all agreed that no one should drink too much, and then as soon as we sat down had ordered champagne, which was currently flowing like water.

'Oh, come on,' said Lisa. 'You know you're dying to find out, Mum. You're just too polite to ask. Be honest, you're glad you've got me to do your dirty work for you. So how did you and Alex meet?'

'Ignore my daughter,' said Cathie, handing me a glass of champagne. 'We already threatened to leave her at home if she didn't behave herself.'

'But I'm chief bridesmaid,' said Lisa indignantly. 'Who is going to keep the rug-rags in line if I'm not here? We only want to know because we love him and we've been trying to get him fixed up for ages. He's way too cute to be on his own.'

Alex laughed, and I'm sure he blushed just a little bit.

'You've got to be something special. He's so bloody picky,' said one of the other girls.

Now it was my turn to redden.

Since waking up Alex and I had shared a shower together, and it would be fair to say that both of us were ravenous, so we had mooted plans to grab a bite to eat and then maybe repeat the afternoon's performance. I had more or less completely forgotten that we were meant to be there for a wedding and so was surprised when, around seven o'clock, someone knocked on our door.

'Helloooo,' called a female voice. 'Alex? Are you in there, darling?'

Alex and I were both still in hotel bathrobes and, having discussed whether it was too early to crack open the mini-bar, were both drinking tea while eating our way through the complimentary biscuits and peanuts and picking over the events of our first afternoon together as Dom and sub.

We had also had a good look at the marks left by the riding crop – in my case in the bathroom mirror. At first Alex had been concerned about them, and asked whether he had hit me too hard. When I said he hadn't and I was fine with them, he was amused and proud by turns about how evenly spaced they were. It had to be a boy thing. He turned me over on the bed onto my stomach and very carefully traced each one with his fingers.

Curled up on the bed together, it was interesting how comfortable I felt with him. Part of me was pleased about that; part of me was wary. I was supposed to be taking this slowly, I reminded myself – although it was probably too late for that.

'Hang on,' Alex called, heading for the door as the woman called again and glancing back over his shoulder towards me, presumably to make sure I was decent. 'You okay?' he mouthed. I nodded. I was more than okay. I plumped up the pillows, poured another cup of tea and helped myself to the last shortbread.

Alex stepped out into a little hallway area that divided the suite from the door to the corridor and pulled the door to behind him, cutting off any view his visitor might have into our room.

'Oh, you are in there,' said a disembodied voice. Whoever it was sounded warm and friendly and genuinely pleased to see him. 'We're all going down to dinner in a little while and wondered if you'd like to come and eat with us.'

'That would be great, thank you, Cathie. We're starving.'

'Good. I'm so glad you could make it.' There was a pause. 'Terry told me that you'd brought a plus one. *We're* starving?' She laughed.

'News travels fast round these parts,' Alex said, though I could hear the amusement in his voice.

'So, do I get to meet her?'

'Last time I saw her she wasn't dressed,' said Alex.

I was glad he had the gumption to keep whoever it was out; I'd rather have my clothes on when I was introduced to his vanilla friends. I glanced round the room; it was strewn with our clothes, not to mention a crop and an open bag with ropes, gags and various other toys in it.

'Oh well, I suppose we'll see her downstairs. I'm glad you've found someone nice, Alex. It's been far too long.'

He laughed. 'What makes you think she's nice?'

The woman laughed too, and from the sound I guessed that she slapped him playfully.

'I'm sure she's lovely. See you in the bar. We said we'd be down at half seven. Is that okay?'

'It's fine. See you down there,' Alex said. 'And it's great to see you, Cathie. You look amazing in that dress.'

'Flatterer,' giggled the woman, evidently delighted with the compliment, and with that Alex closed the door.

\* \* \*

Which was how I came to be sitting next to Lisa on a huge table in among a sea of people I didn't know. Lisa wasn't going to be put off the scent. She might as well have had me under a lamp with thumbscrews.

'We met on a dating website,' I said casually, helping myself to more vegetables. The food was fabulous and I could have eaten a horse – maybe two horses. I'd forgotten that BDSM made me hungry.

'Really?' Lisa pulled a face. 'Online dating? I've never tried it. It can be a bit iffy, can't it?'

'You just have to be sensible and not do anything silly,' I said. Like going away for a weekend with a complete stranger, my brain offered helpfully.

'That's right, and I know lots of people who do it,' said Cathie, not quite meeting anyone's eye. The way she said it made me think that she might be one of them. Apparently the bride's father was a bit of a lad and was driving up the following day with his new wife, number three or four, who was twenty-two. Cathie hadn't brought a plus one, but kept checking her phone, which made me think there was someone in the wings somewhere.

'You read so many things in the papers about all that online stuff – you can meet some seriously weird people,' said the bride's uncle, Harry, who was sitting further around the table.

'Only if you're lucky,' said Alex, lifting a glass towards me in a silent toast.

I smiled. You most certainly could, I thought, as I shuffled my chair in a little closer to the table, trying to ignore the pain from the weals across my bum.

# Chapter Five

Naked except for a black silk ribbon tied into a bow around my neck, and tied down to the huge four-poster bed, all I could see above me were the heavy silk drapes of the bed's ornate canopy and – by turning my head to the left and right – the ornate carving on the bedside cabinets. Not much of a view, and impossible to work out what was going on.

I tested the ropes that secured me to the bed. It was an instinctive response more than any real attempt to escape. Let's face it, I was there with Alex because I wanted to be – I was certainly not being held against my will – but being alone and tied down offers a certain challenge, and if I could untie myself then I most certainly would.

It was our second evening at the hotel for his friend's wedding. The actual wedding had been fabulous, but that wasn't what was on my mind at this particular moment.

I tugged a little harder at the ropes, but not so hard as to tighten the knots. There was no give, which was both gratifying (who wants a Dom who can't tie a decent knot?) and annoying, as I quite liked the idea that when Alex came back I'd be sitting up in bed, naked except for my sweet little black ribbon, a coil of rope and a grin.

I wriggled around to take a look at the way the knots had been tied. The rope securing my wrists had been threaded around behind the bedposts and the headboard, so as I moved it would slip to and fro, and if I eased myself up the bed a little and gave myself a little more slack I was more or less certain that I could undo the knots with my teeth. Alex had very thoughtfully wrapped silk scarves around my wrists and ankles to stop the ropes burning or bruising my skin, but I could still feel the constriction, and the sense of vulnerability and exposure, which all added to the erotic charge that being tied up gave me. An escape attempt was just all part of the game, although I didn't plan to try too hard. I was really pleased to be sharing in the fantasy scenario that had started Alex on the way to embracing the Dom side of his nature.

From outside, through an open window somewhere off to my left, I could hear voices and the sounds of the wedding party in full swing. There were fireworks going off, people laughing and talking, the clink of glasses, the soft strains of a dance band. Inside the suite the air was still and heavy except for the sound of my breathing. I inched a little closer to the edge of the bed and towards one of the knots, imagining my teeth working it loose, pulling it undone, and then wriggling my hand free. It was nylon, a kind of dark-blue woven cord – I could almost taste it.

Slowly, slowly I eased closer and then, opening my mouth, I closed my teeth around one of the strands where it vanished beneath the other and very gently began to pull it free. I closed my eyes, visualising the way the knot was tied. It gave a little and started to loosen just a fraction. I twisted my head. It gave a little more.

'And just what do you think you're doing?' asked an amused voice. 'I obviously can't leave you alone for one minute, can I?'

I opened my eyes and looked up. Alex came over to the side of the bed and into my field of vision. He was still dressed in the crisp white formal shirt and suit trousers he had worn to the wedding and, although he had taken off his jacket and tie, the formal look really suited him. It has to be said that I'm a sucker for a man in a good suit, and he had looked gorgeous in his. I could just see the lightest flurry of chest hair above the open buttons of his shirt. It made me salivate.

The other good news was that he had one arm wrapped around a bottle of champagne in an ice bucket and in his other hand he had two champagne flutes.

'I needed something to do, Sir,' I said, shuffling myself back into the middle of the bed. 'I was getting bored.'

'So I see,' he said. I didn't mention that the rope was now loose enough for me to slip my hand out. 'In that case I think we should find something to take your mind off escaping, don't you?'

'You were the one who just wandered off, Sir,' I said, with mock indignation.

He laughed. In reality Alex had just got me nicely tied up when there had been a knock on the door to our suite. Room service? More friends dropping by? Someone coming to tell us that the bride and groom were about to head off on their honeymoon? I have no idea. Whoever it was, I was in no position to do anything about it. Alex had pulled the bedroom door tight closed behind him this time, and I had heard him chatting away to someone, laughing, make light conversation – although this time I couldn't make out what was being said – for all the world as if he hadn't got a naked woman tied spreadeagled across his bed in the other room. And now he was back. With champagne. Which I couldn't drink because I was tied up.

Alex put the champagne and glasses on the bedside cabinet, then sat down alongside me and took one of the ice cubes from the bucket, his eyes bright with desire and mischief. 'It was Cathie. She thought we might like a bottle to ourselves.'

'Nice of her.'

'And she wanted to know if we were going down.'

'And are we?' I asked.

He grinned. 'We might be. But I'm sure we won't be missed for a while yet. I told her there are a few things I need to take care of first.'

'She seems lovely.'

He nodded. 'She is, but it's not her I want to talk about.' He was quiet and looked me up and down. 'So, where were we?' he asked. 'Oh, I remember. I was going to blindfold you and then have my wicked way with you.' His tone was teasing but with something dark and altogether more exciting lurking just below the surface.

He leaned over me and let a single icy droplet of water drip into the valley between my breasts, making me gasp and shiver. Another drop and my back arched. Alex smiled and leaned in closer still, sliding the icy little gem down over the pit of my throat, circling my breasts and outlining my nipples, and then drawing first one and then the other into his mouth and sucking gently. His warm lips were a sharp contrast to the chilly kiss of the ice cube, which he pressed down onto whichever nipple was not in his mouth. He moaned softly, nipping and gently biting now.

I gasped and closed my eyes, wrapping my hands around the ropes, holding on tight, and then shivered, drinking in the sensations as my nipples stiffened and my skin prickled under his attentions. It felt fabulous and mind-bogglingly intense.

'Oh, that is pretty,' Alex whispered, pulling away and popping what remained of the ice cube into his mouth. I opened my eyes. He was looking down at me, taking in the view.

'I've been thinking about this for such a long time,' he said.

'And?'

'And you look just how I imagined,' he said, as he took a blindfold from the bedside cabinet. Lifting my head from the pillow he slipped the blindfold down over my hair, down over my eyes. 'There we are,' he murmured. 'Perfect.'

For a moment, as I was plunged into darkness, I froze, wondering again if this was such a good idea. Half the fun is *not* seeing what your Dom has planned or is doing, but it also adds to the tension if you don't know them well. This was that crossover moment.

'Are you okay?' Alex murmured gently, stroking my hair. 'If you're unhappy about this we can stop now. Or I can take the blindfold off, if you like. Are you okay?'

I nodded.

'Tell me,' he said. 'I need to hear you say it.'

'I'm okay, Sir,' I said.

'Good girl.'

His lips brushed mine in the lightest and most delicate of kisses, which felt totally at odds with my being tied spreadeagled and naked.

'You look gorgeous. Now, where shall we start?' he said, in a whisper that suggested he was talking to himself.

I waited, my breathing shallow as I listened out for what was coming next. I was expecting pain. Deprived of sight, my senses reached out into the darkness for clues. I could hear dance music and voices from outside and struggled to filter them out so that I could concentrate on Alex. I could hear him moving around the room, unzipping a bag, padding from place to place, but the plush carpet deadened the sounds and made it impossible to work out exactly what he was doing or where exactly he was. And then I felt the mattress give as he got back onto the bed alongside me.

'I've waited so long for this, I've got so many things I want to try,' he whispered. I could hear the arousal and excitement in his voice. I held my breath and braced myself for whatever might follow. To my surprise, instead of the explosive crack of a whip, or a paddle, or the crop, I felt something delicate and incredibly soft brush oh-so-slowly across my skin, starting with my hand, along my arm, into the sensitive valley of my armpit, over my breasts, the other arm, the other hand, then back down over my ribs and stomach, the rise of my sex, my thighs and calves, down across my feet ... A feather? Silk? I'm not sure, but it set my nerve endings tingling with pleasure.

Before I could make up my mind what it was, something nipped at the flesh between neck and breast, hot on the heels of the soft touch. The sensation came rolling down in a continuous line, down over one breast and then on up over the other, then down, down, on over my belly – it felt like a wheel with pins or spikes and made me gasp – and then there was something warm, maybe a warm sponge or cloth, and then ice again. The combinations and contrasts made me shiver and gasp as Alex built up wave after wave of sensation. It was all-engulfing and made my pulse quicken. It felt almost as if Alex was playing me like an instrument, each touch a different note, joining together to form an unlikely chord.

I heard Alex strike a match, and I could pick out the distinctive odour of a candle burning. Though I guessed what was coming next, nothing prepared me for the sensation of hot wax as he dripped it, drop by drop, into the soft pit of my navel. I whimpered and gasped as it hit. It cooled in an instant, landing as a liquid on my flesh but turning to a soft, warm, pliable puddle in seconds. He trickled more, drop by molten drop, up the centre of my body, up over my breastbone, then onto my breasts and collarbones, making me cry out as each little globule dropped, spread and hardened.

Alex followed it up with something rough – perhaps hessian – scouring away the wax, and then something velvety. Then he lightly whipped and flicked at my body with what felt like a fine reed or cane. The sensations were heaped one upon the other and together they were breathtaking. He brought every nerve ending to life with his stroking, his touching, his toying, nipping, pressing, pinching, licking, kissing and heat.

The sounds of the fireworks going off outside in the grounds of the hotel wove themselves into the sensations exploding in my head. My whole body felt as if it was alight, alive, with every molecule of my body and mind glowing and expectant. It felt as if I was submerging into a great sea of pleasure, and then I felt Alex moving slowly down the bed so that he was between my legs.

I waited, imaging what would come next.

He pressed his lips to my navel, circling it, dipping into it with his tongue, kissing every inch of my belly, outlining the bones of my hips with his tongue, kissing the bowl between them and working down to the mound of my sex where he paused and hungrily pressed his nose and lips into the trimmed tangle of my pubic hair, breathing me in, his teeth nipping and biting at the hair.

I moaned and heard myself begging him for more, heard him murmuring his approval as I felt him opening my outer lips with his fingers, felt the very tip of his tongue seeking out my clitoris, circling, sucking, and felt my body opening up like the petals of a flower.

I lifted my hips up off the bed, offering myself to him, wanton and hungry for more of what he had to give me, and he answered my need by licking harder, by sucking, by lapping – I cried out, feeling intense ripples of pleasure wash through me. The pleasure was all-consuming, and as I pressed myself up onto his tongue, I felt something slick, smooth and cool – a dildo, I assumed – pressing insistently at the inner lips of my sex and gasped as Alex guided whatever it was inside me, working it in and out in time with his tongue, which was working its magic on my clitoris. I could feel myself losing control, tipping over into the white raging waters of oblivion, as he pressed on and on.

But just as I got to the very edge, moving my hips in time to his caresses, Alex pulled away.

I gasped, feeling robbed of my prize. 'Please,' I whispered, my voice thick with desire and emotion. 'Please – don't stop now. Please, I'm almost there –'

Alex laughed throatily. 'I love to hear a woman beg,' he said, and then his fingers took the place of this tongue. I gasped as he began to stroke me and work the dildo in and out.

Alex's touch was as informed as his tongue; this was a man who really knew his way around a woman's body. He gently circled the sensitive bud, moving away when it got too intense and when I was almost there, moving back to bring me closer and closer to boiling point, slowly building the intensity, stroke on stroke, edging me closer and closer to orgasm, feeling his way to the boundaries of my pleasure. And each time I got to the brink, he stopped and pulled me back.

The feelings inside me were building and building and building until I could hardly bear it any more. I began to move with him, and now Alex let me dictate the rhythm, let me press myself up onto his fingers and the dildo, until I was stretching up, pulling against the ropes. And then suddenly I was there, teetering on the brink of no return. The next circling brush of his fingers and I tumbled headlong into the swelling, boiling mass of orgasm, gasping, sobbing, galvanised by the sheer intensity of the pleasure he had given me, bucking and writhing under his knowing touch.

I was astonished as I came and came and came; something that had never happened to me before. Even as I thrust upwards enjoying the last vestiges of pleasure, there was a part of me that was very conscious of Alex watching me come, exposed and hungry, and while part of me felt ashamed of my wanton need, the rest of me didn't care. Finally, exhausted, I fell back among the tumble of pillows. As I lay there shivering with the aftershocks of orgasm, I felt Alex remove whatever it was that had been inside me and instead slide in between my legs.

As he moved into position I felt the very tip of his cock brushing the tender skin inside my thighs, eager to be inside me, eager to meet his own needs and to bring this exquisite dance to its conclusion. His manhood was engorged and hungry as he pressed home into the swollen, sensitised depths of my sex.

I called out in pure pleasure as Alex drove into me, my body opening for him as he thrust deeper and deeper, ferocious now and with a raging hunger that my body was only too happy to satisfy. I lifted my pelvis up to meet his; I wanted more than anything to share and repay the pleasure he had given me and thrust up to meet his next stroke. I heard him gasp as I flexed my muscles deep inside and my sex tightened around him, hot and wet and still throbbing from orgasm.

'Lie still,' Alex ordered, his voice dark and throaty now as he pushed me down hard onto the bed. As he brought his face closer to mine I could feel his breath on my cheek and pick out the scent of my body lingering on his lips.

'Just lie very still,' he said, when I moaned in protest. 'I want you to feel me. Just feel me – let me take you – let me –'

Against the odds, and the instinctive reaction of my body to his movements, I did as I was told. And then Alex found his rhythm, pressing deep, in and out, taking his time, giving us both time to savour the feeling as he moved against me. I couldn't remember a time when I had ever lain still during sex, but there was something strangely thrilling in feeling him, really feeling, concentrating on the sensation of penetration and him moving deep inside, feeling my body close around him, taking him deeper, and at the same time knowing that it was bringing him closer and closer to the brink.

My whole body ached to echo his thrust. I longed to join him in the dance that would see him come, but I did as I was told and moaned with pure pleasure as I heard the breath catch in his throat, heard a dark, hungry groan from deep in his chest. Then his movements quickened and I could hold back no longer. I lifted my hips to meet his and he pushed deeper still – so deep that he took my breath away. We moved as one and it seemed like we went on and on and on until suddenly, deep, deep inside, I felt his cock pulsing, again and again, as he came.

Alex cried out, gasping and moaning, and then all at once he was done and collapsed down on top of me as if he had been shot. In the moments that followed we both lay still, both struggling for breath, both hot and sweating and breathing hard, both spent, both completely consumed and burnt up by pleasure. After a few seconds Alex pressed kisses into my neck, sliding the blindfold up over my hair.

I blinked as my eyes adjusted to the lamplight and I made the effort to focus, while Alex, his hair tousled and a bead of sweat running down his temple, turned his attention to the ropes that still bound me to the bed frame.

As our eyes met, he smiled.

'Was that what you had hoped for, Sir?' I asked.

His smiled widened into a lazy grin. 'It was perfect.' And then he reached out and touched the black ribbon that was still tied around my neck. 'You look good in a collar. I want you to keep this on when we go downstairs.'

'So we are going downstairs?' I asked.

He nodded. 'It would be rude not to. And besides, Cathie only gave me the champagne on condition that we came down and danced with her and the girls later.'

I laughed. 'I'll be lucky if I can walk, let alone dance.'

Alex grinned and unfastened my ankles. Once he had untied the ropes he settled himself on the bed alongside me, put an arm around my shoulders, holding me tight up against him, and pulled a throw over us. It felt good.

Instinctively I nuzzled into his chest, feeling safe and warm in his arms.

He smelt good, a subtle mixture of warm masculinity and sex. It felt nice to be there with him and so very good to be playing again. As we started to doze he pulled me in closer still so that the hair on his chest brushed my chin and I could hear the strong rhythmic beat of his heart.

'That was wonderful,' he murmured. 'I'm really glad you said that you'd come.'

'Me too,' I said. 'What time did you tell Cathie we would be downstairs?'

'Oh, we're okay. I told her we'd be down later on.'

'Really? And what reason did you give her?'

Alex laughed. 'I told her that I'd got you tied to the bed and that we might be some time.'

I pushed myself up onto one elbow and stared at him. 'You didn't really say that, did you?'

He grinned. 'Actually I did, and Cathie just laughed and said, "Right, well, in that case don't let me stop you. You'd better get back to her." I'm assuming she thought I was joking, or maybe she is a lot more broadminded than I thought.'

I stared at him.

'Do you fancy a glass of champagne?' he asked, nodding towards the ice bucket.

I nodded, although I would have preferred to go to sleep.

He poured us both a glass. 'Have you given any thought to staying for an extra night? We could go out tomorrow and see a few of the sights, and then drive back on Sunday.'

I hesitated. 'It would be nice but –'

'But you need to be getting back?'

I was about to nod and agree, because it was the sensible thing to do, but then I thought about what I really felt and what I really wanted and instead said: 'Oh, what the hell. Actually I'd love to stay another night. It would be nice to take a look around now we're here. We've barely been out of the hotel.'

Alex laughed. 'Oh, and that's been a problem, has it?'

Hard not to smile. 'Hardly,' I said.

'Okay. Well, in that case let me just ring down to reception.'

'Thank you,' I said, taking a sip from my glass. 'I've had a really nice time.'

'You make it sound like a trip to the zoo.'

I laughed. 'Sorry, but it's been a great weekend.'

'For me too,' said Alex. 'And hopefully it won't be the last.'

I said nothing.

Once Alex had confirmed we could have the suite for another night, we got up, showered, dressed and went down to join the others for the evening party. Strangely enough, I felt like I could have danced all night.


The following day, once the wedding party had said their farewells over breakfast and Alex had sworn that, yes, he would bring me up to stay at Cathie's for the weekend and that, yes, we had had the most fabulous time, Alex and I set off on the tourist trail.

It was bliss. We spent the whole day exploring Whitby, wandering around the fabulous old town on the far side of the River Esk, walking out on the harbour wall, visiting the abbey and then driving on to Robin Hood's Bay before finally, in homage to our first date, having a fish-and-chip supper in one of Whitby's famous fish restaurants.

By the time we got back to the hotel we were both exhausted. Curled up in each other's arms, we fell sound asleep within minutes of climbing into bed.

When I woke up, still in Alex's arms, on Sunday morning I couldn't think of anywhere I would rather be. Over breakfast we both agreed that it would be nice to have more time, to come back and explore some more, and when I said it I truly meant it. We drove home on Sunday morning, taking our time, stopping for lunch en route and generally just enjoying each other's company. The truth was I'd had the best time and was quite sad that it was over.

As we pulled into a parking space outside my place, Alex said: 'Thank you for the most fabulous weekend. I've had a great time.'

'Me too,' I said. 'Thank you for inviting me. It was really good fun.'

He looked at me with a question in his expression.

'What?' I laughed. 'Would you like to come in and have a coffee before you go?'

He shook his head. 'No, I'd better be getting back. I just thought you were going to say "but …"'

'No, I wasn't.'

He smiled. There was something in his face that made me think there was more he wanted to say.

'What is it?'

He held my gaze. 'Can we try this? You and me. Dom and sub.'

I hesitated. Part of me was certain it would work; part of me was cynical, hurt and terrified of making another big mistake. What if I'd got it wrong? What were the odds of this being the right relationship for me, straight out of the trap?

'Alex,' I said. 'I've had the best time.'

He stared at me. 'But?'

'No, no buts. I have really enjoyed myself. It's been brilliant.'

'So when can I see you again?'

Sometimes the only thing to say is the truth. 'What if this is me on the rebound?' I asked.

Alex pulled a face. 'I'm not with you.'

'I really have had the most fabulous time, and being with you feels right, and I think you're lovely.' I knew I was talking too much – and that I was giving good reasons to carry on, not good reasons to stop – but I couldn't stop myself.

'I'm not with you,' Alex said again. 'You're making it sound like all those are bad things?'

'Well, they might be. No, I mean, I know they're not, but I'm worried about hurting you and hurting me.' I paused, feeling bewildered. God only knows what Alex was thinking. 'I'm not sure I'm ready for a thing,' I said in desperation.

Alex laughed. 'A *thing*? What sort of a thing?'

'A relationship. That's what you want, isn't it?'

He nodded. 'Yes, I do, and I was rather hoping I could have one with you.'

'But what if we're wrong, what if *I'm* wrong. What if it's too soon – too fast?'

'This from the woman who I spent the weekend beating and tying to the bed on the strength of a chip supper and an ice cream?' he said wryly.

I nodded.

'So what if it is? Does it matter? We could try it out and see how we get on. How does that sound?'

I slumped back in the seat, wishing he had taken me up on my invitation to come in so we could be having this conversation over a pot of tea in the kitchen, taking our time, not rushing it. But there was also a part of me that knew if we went into the house we'd end up in bed together.

'I fell in love with Max,' I said.

Alex nodded. 'I know, you told me.'

'In some ways I feel like I'm still about fifteen when it comes to all this relationship stuff. I got married early; I never really experimented.'

'You seem to be doing okay now,' he laughed.

I nodded. 'And I think that's just it. That's the problem. I'm doing what I should have done in my teens and twenties, Alex, and looking back now I'm not sure if I fell in love with Max for who he was or the things that he offered me.'

'BDSM?'

I nodded. 'And romance and adventure and doing things I'd always dreamed about and never thought I'd get around to doing. I promised myself that if there was a next time I would take it more slowly.'

'Which means what exactly?' he asked. 'Given that we've just had a brilliant weekend away together.'

I shook my head. 'I don't know really. I'm just afraid of getting hurt all over again or hurting you. You're far too nice to hurt.'

He grinned. 'I'm a big boy, Sarah. I can take care of myself.'

I nodded. 'I know.'

'You're serious, aren't you?'

I nodded again, feeling my eyes fill up with unexpected tears. 'I'm nervous about wrecking everything and getting it all wrong again. I want to be with the right person.'

'I think that's me,' Alex said, suddenly serious. 'I thought that as soon as we met.'

I knew he was right because I had felt it too, but that worried me even more. 'Even if I feel like that too, Alex, it's way too soon.'

'So what do you suggest?' he said 'That we just ignore it, chalk it up to experience and go our separate ways?'

That wasn't what I wanted at all but what choice had I given him? I slumped down into the seat. 'I don't know. I don't know what I want.'

'Okay, I'll tell you what, let's do what you said, let's take it slow. We don't have to commit to anything or anyone. Do whatever you feel it is you need to do to sort this out in your head, and then in six months' time we'll both see how we feel.'

I stared at him. 'Seriously?'

He nodded. 'I'm happy to wait for six months.'

I stared at him. 'Wait?'

'I've waited for a long time to get to this point and I think you're worth waiting for, Sarah. And I'm not in a muddle about how I feel. Yes, it's early days; no, I don't want to get hurt either, but I'm prepared to take a risk. Just don't leave it too long. And let's get this perfectly straight: it's a one-time only deal. You only get one shot at this. I'm not going to wait around forever. Six months and then we decide. Take it or leave it.'

'Really?'

He nodded. 'And I think I could do with that tea now.'

As we got out of the car and he was getting my case out of the boot I said: 'And I think you should know that I've put my profile back on the website.'

He nodded, without so much as breaking his stride. 'That's fine,' he said.

'Fine?' I said.

Apparently unfazed, he nodded.

I reddened. 'I can explain,' I said.

'There's no need. Let's go inside and get the kettle on,' Alex said.

So we did, and I was right about us ending up in bed.

# Chapter Six

No, I hadn't told Alex that before we had headed north to Whitby I had put my profile back up on the BDSM website. Sounds mad? Sounds duplicitous? I know, but it wasn't really meant to be either. I saw it as insurance in case our trip away was a disaster or, maybe worse still, that it wasn't. I'd been married for so long before embarking on a single life that my dating and relationship skills, despite the BDSM twist, felt to me as if they were stuck in a time warp.

I needed to remind myself that there was no need to rush, no need to panic; there were plenty more fish in the sea and I didn't have to fall for the first one I pulled out of the net. After all these years of longing for a taste of BDSM, didn't it make sense to explore a little more before settling down into a long-term relationship with someone?

Once Alex had finally left and I had unpacked, collected the dog from the kennels and tracked down the cats, who had been fed by my next-door neighbour while I was away, I switched on my computer and picked up my emails. To keep my everyday and business life separate from BDSM (and to safeguard against the faint but nonetheless real possibility that one of my children, albeit my grown-up children, might use my computer or laptop), I had a separate email account for the site, one that meant I had to go online to pick up the mail. Things had been busy in my absence. I had an inbox full of replies to my ad.

This is not an exaggeration, nor is it about being in any way super-attractive or my ad being super-explicit; there are generally far fewer women on BDSM websites than men. I'm not sure if this is because men are more into Ds and more upfront about their sexual tastes, or more eager or confident about turning their fantasies into reality, or perhaps because women are more reluctant to advertise their desires or have very reasonable concerns about being vulnerable to abuse and are therefore anxious that they might be putting themselves at risk. Whatever the reason, it means that as a woman you get a lot of attention.

While having so many emails is flattering, it's been obvious to me ever since I advertised the first time that a large number of the men on the site adopt a scattergun approach to finding a partner and will email anything with a pulse with what is obviously a bog-standard email. Halfway through the first line it is blindingly apparent that they haven't read your profile. The different tones also take some getting used to. Some men take the role-playing aspect to the extreme and write like a despotic emperor; some are just very crude; some write as if they're back in the Middle Ages – though personally I have zero tolerance for being addressed as 'wench' – some are badly spelt and coarse, so the replies generally take some weeding through before you find people you may be interested in getting to know better.

You also get a lot of one-liners – some even in text speak – commenting on your appearance (if you've posted a photo): 'You've got nice <insert body part of choice>.' Sometimes they were blatantly offering sex. I did wonder, reading the various and sometimes very graphic suggestions, if anyone ever replied to them. 'Dear Mr Horny-Toad, Thank you for your email. I'd love to take you up on your offer of a shag/extraordinary sexual suggestion/deviation/illegal act.'

But it wouldn't be me answering their emails. I may be confused and muddled when it comes to choosing and then negotiating my way round a relationship, but I'm not desperate, and I do like a man who has more to offer than the ability to type 'RU up 4 it?'

The phone rang as I was sifting the wheat from the chaff. At first I thought it was Alex, phoning to let me know he had got home safely, and then realised I was disappointed when it wasn't.

It was Gabbie. 'And?' she said, by way of a greeting.

'And it was lovely. We had a great time.'

'And are you seeing him again?'

'Very possibly.' Despite imposing the six-month rule on getting seriously involved with each other, we had both agreed that we would still like to keep in touch, see each other, maybe go out once in a while, maybe sleep together, maybe have him tie me up and whip me 'til I begged him to stop – after all, why waste a talent like his? It was a whole new twist on friends with benefits. BDSM benefits.

There was no disputing that what we had enjoyed over the weekend was good. Better than good.

'We're just going to take it slow,' I said, while deleting an email where the only content was a grainy photo of an erect male member, taken from above, and which hadn't been that much to write home about before he tied a ribbon round it. How would you recognise this man in the pub?

'So he wasn't that great?' suggested Gabbie.

'Alex?' My mind wasn't fully on the conversation.

'Yes, who else would I be talking about?'

I sighed, my eyes still on the computer screen. The next email was from a man whose wife didn't understand him, but who wouldn't mind him tying up women as long as she didn't find out. I turned my full attention to Gabbie.

'Sorry,' I said, closing the lid on my laptop. 'I was just sorting out some stuff on the computer. Alex was better than great. I had a fabulous time. Whitby is just amazing – and Alex is good company, he really made me laugh. He's great in bed. His friends love him, and I wish we'd had more time together. It was about as close to perfect as any date I've ever been on.'

'Well, for God's sake. What is your problem?'

'What if I'm making it up? What if I'm imagining it? What if I'm wrong?'

'Oh, please,' snapped Gabbie.

'I'm serious. The thing with Max took me so long to get over –'

'I know, sweetie.'

'I know I wanted to lose a few pounds but the misery diet really isn't one I'd recommend. This thing with Alex might just be lust.'

'There's nothing wrong with a bit of good old-fashioned lust.'

'Which is what we've both more or less agreed on, and in which case it will burn out. It's just that he wants a thing.'

'A *thing*?'

'A relationship.'

'And you don't?'

'Of course I do, but I don't want to be in the wrong one, or to start one that's going nowhere or to hurt him. Or me. I'm scared.'

'You think too much. Sometimes you have to just try. It's what we all do. Sometimes these things work, sometimes they don't. It's what being human is all about. He sounds lovely –'

'He is. I'm just trying, for once, to let my head rule my heart, not get involved, take it slowly and just see what happens.'

Gabbie laughed. 'Okay, honey, well, good luck with that. Anyway, besides ringing up to see how you'd got on, I rang to tell you that Helen called me and said it was high time we all got together and had supper.'

'I've been saying that for weeks.'

'I know, but now everyone is saying it, so it's happening. My place. I was thinking maybe Moroccan, couscous, orange water and tagines? What do you think?'

'I can hardly wait,' I said. And I meant it. It had been far too long since we'd all got together.

'I'll email round some dates.'

'Brilliant.'

'And then you can tell us all about why you're not going to have a relationship with Alex,' she said, laughter bubbling up.

'Bugger off,' I said.

And with that, and still laughing, Gabbie hung up and I turned my attention back to my inbox.

# Chapter Seven

The lamb, slow-cooked with pine nuts and apricots, was a masterpiece. I'd brought along a minced beef dish that I'd found online, cooked with lots of spices and served in warm pitta pockets with a blob of yoghurt and a sprinkling of chilli as a garnish, along with a zillion-calories-a-portion dessert that I'd found in a Sunday colour supplement. Joan had brought bowls of amazing salads, couscous and flatbreads, and Helen had brought breakfast. We were eating our Moroccan feast by lamplight in front of a roaring log fire, sitting around a coffee table on the floor on big cushions as an homage to the whole North African theme.

As it had been a while since we'd all seen each other we'd planned a sleepover. Everyone had brought wine and duvets and pjs and was looking forward to a long, lazy evening and a long lie-in. It felt like the best kind of get-together and we'd done nothing but talk since we'd all arrived.

Gabbie had got us a girlie DVD, although we all had so much catching up to do chances were it would go unwatched. Tradition had it that we didn't usually talk about the big things in our lives or our families until we were all together, all eating or had eaten and everyone could hear, so that we could all comment and join in.

'So,' said Gabbie, tapping on the side of a glass as we finished off the remains of the main course, 'I'd really like to propose a toast to the four of us: all still here, all still friends and all still crazy after all these years.'

Joan pulled a face. 'You speak for yourself.'

Helen laughed and we all clinked glasses with gusto. 'Hear, hear!' she said. It had to be said that Helen looked amazing. Since the last time I'd seen her she had lost weight, and looked as if she had given her wardrobe a makeover and done something different with her hair, which was now shorter, lighter and feathered – it took years off her. 'Anyway, I've got an announcement to make,' she said, with a beaming smile. 'I've been dying to tell you.'

We all turned to look at her. We had barely seen each other for the last few months, and though it didn't take long for us to catch up once we were all together, sitting round the table laughing and chatting with them made me realise just how much I'd missed them all. And during those months some of our fundamental rules had gone by the by, like getting together to vet each other's new men, and the day-to-day things that bound us together had been overlooked. I think we had all missed the support of meeting up regularly. Emails and phone calls were a poor substitute.

'Me too,' said Joan, pouring herself another glass of wine.

We all turned to look at her. 'You first,' she said to Helen, waving her into action.

'No, you,' said Helen. 'You can't do that. Just say you've got an announcement and say nothing. Everyone knows everything about me. And what they don't know they can guess.'

I suspected neither of them wanted to be the also-ran in the announcement stakes, but Joan held firm. 'Okay,' said Helen finally, unable to help herself. 'Geoff has asked me to move in with him!' She practically squealed the last few words.

'Wow!' said Gabbie, eyes widening. 'All a bit sudden, isn't it? Whatever happened to what's-his-name?'

'Rob,' said Joan. 'The nice one.'

'And what do any of us know about this Geoff, eh?' I added.

'Nothing,' said Gabbie, playing along. 'Because none of us has met him.'

Aping offence, all three of us turned to stare at her in unison. Helen laughed. 'Play nicely, you lot. You will meet him, I promise. We just haven't sorted out quite when yet.'

'Well, you'd better be quick,' said Joan. 'We really ought to meet him before you move in together. Just in case.'

'Have you said yes?' Gabbie asked. It was obvious from Helen's expression that she had and that she was happy with her decision, but that didn't mean we were, or that we couldn't tease her.

'She can't. We haven't met him; you know the rules,' I said, trying to look disapproving and failing miserably.

'I know, I know, and yes, I do know the rules, so we're having a bit of a party at my place in the summer and I want you all to come. He's lovely,' purred Helen. 'And he's dying to meet you all. He's a bit quiet when you first meet him but he's so sweet and great with the kids and he's really good around the house.' She pulled out her phone, flicked through the images and handed it to Gabbie, who peered at the screen and made a noise of approval.

'You make him sound like a Labrador,' she said.

'He's really kind,' Helen gushed. 'We met when he came over to do some work on the house. He's really good with his hands –'

'*Really?*' asked Joan, adding in a little hint of naughtiness. 'When you say *really* good ...?' She left the question hanging, dripping with suggestiveness, and we all laughed.

'And that too,' said Helen, lifting her eyebrows. 'And not just with his hands, either.'

There was an awful lot more good-humoured teasing and Helen was grinning like a loon. 'So what do you think?' she said, nodding towards the picture on the phone.

I glanced at the screen. It was a shot of the two of them at a party. Helen, wrapped in a pashmina, was leaning up against a man. She was looking fabulous and glowing and all loved up. And Geoff? I'm not sure how much you can really tell from a photo, but we all try, don't we? Geoff looked okay; he was smiling, dressed in a checked shirt, and was balding, in his late forties and a bit overweight. If

I'm honest, he looked a bit bland and ordinary, whereas I don't see Helen as ordinary at all. I always imagined her with someone special, because to me she is special. I was sure he was nice. I hoped he was nice.

'What does he do?' I asked, handing the phone on.

'Carpenter,' she said, as Joan put on her reading glasses to take a long, hard look at the screen. 'He's widowed, got his own business. His kids are grown up. He's got a boy and a girl. And he's renovating a house in the village next to mine.'

'So you'll be moving into *his* house, will you?' asked Gabbie, raising her eyebrows.

'Well, yes, but he didn't live there with his family. It's more or less a clean sheet, and I'm going to rent mine out for six months, just to see how we get on, and then we'll think about what comes next.'

Gabbie nodded. 'Fair enough, sounds sensible. Although we have to meet him, obviously.'

'Obviously, and you will. He's really looking forward to meeting you lot. I've told him all about you.'

'Bloody hell, and he still wants to meet us?' said Gabbie.

Helen nodded. 'He's been living in a mobile home on site while he's been doing his house up. And while it was so cold over the winter he spent a lot of time at my place.'

'Cosy,' said Joan, who up until now hadn't said very much at all.

'It has been,' said Helen, sounding defensive. 'And it's been lovely. We've really got to know each other and we've been planning what we're going to do with the inside of his place – our place – and what we're going to do to the garden. Buying things, planning colours ...' Her voice tailed off.

'That sounds absolutely lovely,' I said. 'I'm envious.'

I didn't want her to feel that we were somehow disappointed or disapproving. We *were* all pleased for her, it was just that we had all been through so much together and all been resolutely single for so long. Men had come and gone but our friendship hadn't wavered. It had always been there at the core of our lives. None of us had had anything more than a semi-permanent relationship since we split up from our respective husbands, and I think at some level we all feared that if one of us settled down the friendship we had would change and maybe get lost. So this wasn't just a big step for Helen, it was a big step for all of us.

'You'll still be able to come to the get-togethers, won't you?' I asked.

'Of course I will,' she laughed. 'I wouldn't give up you lot for the world.'

I held up my glass. 'Good,' I said. 'Because otherwise he would have to go.'

Helen laughed. 'I've already told him that you lot are non-negotiable.'

'As long as that's absolutely clear then,' Gabbie said. 'I hope you are really, really happy together, and we can't wait to meet him, can we, ladies?' There was a murmur of agreement. 'I think this deserves another toast.'

We all filled our glasses.

'And we want to come and see the house,' said Joan. 'And the garden.'

'Oh God, yes,' said Gabbie. 'We want to hear *all* about it.'

'And see photos,' said Joan.

'I was going to bring the plans over but I thought that was a bit premature,' said Helen.

'It's a shame you don't live closer. I could do with a good carpenter,' said Gabbie.

'You just want someone who is good with their hands,' teased Joan.

'So,' said Helen, after a few more minutes of toing and froing about how wonderful Geoff was and drinking a toast and talking about how nice the house was and their ideas for the inside and the garden, 'that's my news. What about you, Joan? What were you going to tell us?'

Joan, who was topping up her wine glass for another round, sighed and for one horrible moment I thought she was going to tell us she was ill. Then she said: 'I'm getting married.'

Talk about a bombshell. We all stared at her.

'No,' said Gabbie in astonishment, finally breaking the silence. 'You can't be.'

'Well, I am,' said Joan. She leaned across the table to pick up her bag. 'I've got your invitations in here somewhere.'

'You can't just leave it at that,' said Gabbie. 'You have to tell us everything.'

We all nodded. 'Bloody hell,' said Helen. 'How could you keep that one quiet?'

Joan had had a long and tricky marriage to a grumpy man who in the end had run away with a younger woman.

Eventually, he had wanted to come back and had been livid when Joan wouldn't let him.

He had broken Joan's big soft heart. It had been messy. I had always thought that, of all of us, Joan was the least likely to remarry. Since the split she had got very involved in her local church and eventually became a deacon. She had never, ever mentioned that she was seeing anyone and seemed far keener on work, God and her two fox terriers than dating.

'You didn't even tell us you were seeing someone. You know the rules,' said Helen.

'You can talk,' said Joan, continuing to root around in her bag.

'Yes, but I *did* tell you I was seeing someone.'

'Yes, but we haven't met him,' said Joan, as she finally pulled out three envelopes and handed them round.

I turned the envelope over, slipped my finger under the flap and slid out the cream card. Inside, on beautiful, understated wedding stationery, it seemed that Joan and Tom requested the pleasure of my company and anyone else I'd like to bring, to celebrate the occasion of their wedding and join them at a party afterwards.

'Tom?' said Gabbie, taking the word right out of my mouth. 'Is he someone you met at church?'

Joan, as I said, was a deacon.

'Good Lord, no,' said Joan. 'No, I met him at work. He came in to buy a present for a friend.'

'Have you got a photo?' asked Gabbie.

'Of the present?' asked Joan incredulously.

Gabbie sniffed. 'Very clever. No, not of the present, daft – of Tom. The man you're going to marry.'

'No, I haven't.'

'But you're getting married,' protested Gabbie. 'You can't show up here telling us that you're going to get married and not have a photo. What if we don't approve? What if his face doesn't fit? You know the rules.'

Joan smiled. 'I did think about bringing one, but it's a funny thing and something I never thought I'd say, but I don't really mind what you think of him. I know he's the one. He's fat and funny and he cooks and likes music and the dogs, and I was going to bring a photo but the thing is I'm absolutely certain that I'm doing the right thing. I don't need your approval, because it feels absolutely the right thing to do.'

Gabbie, for once, was totally speechless.

I stared at Joan. She might not have undergone the transformation that Helen had, but there was definitely a twinkle in her eyes, and maybe it was all together healthier. Whoever this Tom was, she didn't feel the need to change herself for him.

'Oh my God,' said Gabbie finally, looking at me. 'And then there were two.'

At which point my phone beeped to announce an incoming text message, and Gabbie rolled her eyes. 'Don't tell me it's lover boy. Make that: and then there was one.'

'You too?' said Helen eagerly, looking straight at me.

'No. And he's not *lover boy*,' I hissed. 'He's not anything at the moment. Okay?'

'At least not for six months,' Gabbie said to the others. 'She's keeping him on hold, on a sort of trial basis.'

Ignoring the three of them, I pulled out the phone. Gabbie was right. It was Alex. The text read: 'Hope you and the girls are having a great time. I've got a chance to get some tickets for an outdoor concert in the summer. Do you fancy it and do you want to ask your gang if they want to come along too?'

There were a few details underneath and the headline act was someone we all loved; it was tempting, and I quite liked the idea of them meeting him. It chimed with the whole let's-be-friends vibe that I was trying to keep between us.

'And?' said Gabbie.

I handed her the phone. She scrolled down. 'He signed it: "Hope to see you soon, love A."'

'Not that, Gabbie. Do you want to go to the concert?'

'What man? What concert?' asked Helen, taking the phone. 'Have you got a picture of him on here?'

'No,' I said.

Joan laughed. 'Come on, you know how they feel about photos.'

'And you know the rules about new men,' added Helen.

'Oh come off it, you two can talk,' I protested. 'And anyway, he isn't a new man. He's just a friend.'

'A friend who took her away for a dirty weekend. And who is very good in bed and –'

I glared at Gabbie. 'Well, thanks for keeping that to yourself,' I snapped. 'It's nothing serious, okay? I'm just taking it slowly. Keeping my options open.'

'Shopping around; playing the field,' added Gabbie, and she was right, I was. I had trawled through the replies I'd had to my advert on the BDSM website and had started to talk to some of the Doms who had replied, both by email and by phone – not that I planned to share that with Helen, Joan and Gabbie.

Something else had happened too. Among the pile of emails I had in my inbox when I got home from Whitby was one from the editor of an erotic imprint who over the years I had written several books for. We got on really well and he would mail from time to time to ask if I had another book in the pipeline.

For the last few years I'd been concentrating on writing romance so, although I loved working with him, up until now I had said no. But it seemed to me that now was the perfect moment to explore and write some more. Now I had the courage and the experience to play if I wanted to and just talk if I didn't. I had more to say about the BDSM experience, simply because I knew more. And contacting the new flush of Doms? It occurred to me that if it didn't work out then I could just put it all down to research. So I had emailed my editor back and said that I might well have something for him, if he could wait just a little while longer.

'So,' said Gabbie, lifting her glass in the second toast of the evening, 'here's to weddings and people moving in and people keeping their options open.'

'I'll drink to that,' I said.

# Chapter Eight

I'd arranged to meet Gareth in London, in Chinatown. In his reply to my personal ad he'd said he was looking for a regular partner to play with, but was absolutely emphatic that he didn't see any emotional or romantic relationship developing beyond play. He preferred to have an exclusive relationship with this partner, and was happy to be friends, but said he also understood that might not be possible.

Given that I'd just bucked at the idea of having a proper ongoing relationship with Alex, I decided to meet him – that, and the fact that he was well over six foot tall, extremely handsome, had a lovely voice and wrote a cracking email.

Coming round the corner off Shaftesbury Avenue, Gareth cut quite a dash in a long duster coat and chocolate-brown fedora. When he spotted me he smiled and doffed it like some leading man in a 1930s spy thriller. It was hard not to be impressed as we said our hellos and he took my arm and we headed off to eat.

'The thing is,' Gareth said over lunch, 'I've been on my own since I was in my late teens. It's not that I'm incapable of loving someone – I've had relationships in the past. It's just that I prefer my own space and I'm not sure anyone can sustain the intensity of the kind of relationships you and I prefer in a domestic setting.' As we were in a very public place, I appreciated that he was choosing his words carefully, and it was the same sentiment that had been expressed by Max on numerous occasions. While in a perfect world I wanted both, given that I'd turned that possibility down maybe this was the way forward until I could find what I was truly looking for.

'And to be frank,' Gareth continued, 'I need that aspect far more than I need someone to cook and clean for me or do my washing. You do understand, don't you?'

I nodded. *That aspect* being a penchant for BDSM.

'Lots of women seem to think that they can bring me round eventually or that I'm lying or that if I only spend time with them I will change my mind, but I can assure you that is not the case. So, if you're looking for a boyfriend or husband, I'm afraid I'm really not your man,' Gareth said, with a wry smile.

I nodded. We had talked about this before meeting, but he obviously felt the need to remind me now that we were face to face.

'I grew up helping to run the family farm with my mother and father, and as soon as I was able to I moved into one of the farm cottages. I have lived on my own ever since. When my parents died I had the main house refurbished and I live there now, on my own. And I'm perfectly fine.'

I nodded.

Gareth was charming, an ex-public school boy, with a dignified, reserved demeanour and impeccable manners. To disguise a receding hairline he had shaved his head, which, with his dark eyes, long lashes and healthy tan, made him look more like a pirate or even a priest than a farmer.

Like Max, Gareth was into old-school BDSM, taking a very formal approach to his relationship with his submissives. He had already emailed to let me know that if we played he would need me to sign a contract, and to help me make up my mind he had already sent me a draft copy to look through. He also expected his submissives to dress as he instructed and to refer to him as Sir or Master while in his presence. This was familiar territory, and the rules that Max liked to play by.

Today, for our first meeting, I was wearing a smart pencil skirt and jacket with a crisp white blouse that opened down the front, a string of pearls and matching earrings, along with stockings and suspenders, low navy court shoes, no knickers and a front-fastening bra. The thinking behind this – besides Gareth having what I suspected might be a prim-but-horny-secretary fantasy – was that in theory, as a submissive, my body was available for him to use whenever he chose to make use of it.

Realistically I had no intention of being available to Gareth unless the fancy took me, but the mind-set of being submissive and obeying the rules set down by the Dom is such an important component of Ds that dressing as instructed and the notion of being available adds a little frisson to any encounter. It is part of playing the complex game of BDSM.

After some discussion by email and on the phone, Gareth had suggested that we meet up in London and go to the theatre, which was a first and made a nice change from meeting up in pubs and eateries. I'd travelled into the city by train and the plan was to have lunch and then catch a matinée performance of *Les Misérables* – his idea, not mine. We were currently eating Chinese food in an all-you-can-eat buffet, which, while it wasn't exactly fine dining, was fun and nicely contrary for a first meeting.

'The other thing is that I don't anticipate having full intercourse with anyone,' Gareth said, guiding a sliver of chicken into his mouth with chopsticks. He had ordered a glass of wine for me and a glass of water for himself, explaining that he didn't drink alcohol but didn't mind if I did. It was a bit of a showstopper – the sex thing, that is, not the teetotalism – after what had been a pretty good opening to a first meeting.

'Really?' I said, through a mouthful of egg noodles. 'What, not at all?'

He nodded.

I couldn't quite believe it, but I decided to press on. The table behind us was full of Chinese tourists chattering away nineteen to the dozen. If they understood what was being said they gave no sign of it. As for going slowly on taking a Ds relationship from play to full sex, I'd been there before too, although with Max it had been me who had wanted to wait until I knew him better before we had sex. Maybe what Gareth really meant was that he just needed time.

Gareth smiled. 'I can see you think I'm open to persuasion, but sex is not on the menu, nor any unnecessary nudity.'

*Unnecessary nudity?* I nearly choked, but I could see from his expression that he was being absolutely serious.

'When I was younger I was involved in an accident and I am unable to have intercourse, and before you say, "Yes, but there are creams, pills, surgery, pumps, injections and God knows what else," I know all about them, but what you need to understand is that I've found a way to satisfy my sexual needs that suits me very well.' The smile held. 'And before you have me down as some sort of sad, repressed loony, I'm not dysfunctional in any other way. I am very happy with who I am, and what I am capable of, but if you want to play then you need to be aware that there will be no sex and I won't be the one getting naked.'

I stared at him.

'And by the way, I love your outfit,' he said, lifting a prawn cracker towards me, in lieu of a toast presumably.

'Really?' I said.

He laughed. 'Really. And don't worry, I'm very good at what I do – I've had no complaints so far.'

Okay, so I was curious, and yes, attracted to him too, which was why the following week I found myself driving out to Gareth's house, in the middle of nowhere, dressed in my best secretarial get-up, with painted nails, a pair of sky-high heels on the passenger seat and tortoiseshell-framed glasses tucked into my retro handbag. A big part of Ds for me was the fun of playing dress-up.

Daft? Possibly, but he was one of the first Doms on my list and he had taken the unprecedented step of getting an ex-sub of his to email me and then, after we'd exchanged a few emails, to ring me to vouch for him, his sanity and trustworthiness.

'Gareth is a total angel,' the woman said. She had a clipped cut-glass accent to match his and had given me her home phone number to ring so that I could check her out. 'He and I were involved with each other for a couple of years, and he is very, very good at what he does. We had a fabulous time, but at the end of the day, darling – and I know he won't mind me telling you this because we parted as good friends – I needed more than what was on offer, and he wasn't prepared to give it. He told you about his accident? And the rules?'

'No sex, no nudity?'

'Those are the ones. Well, to begin with I thought he might be joking or that eventually he might thaw out, but they are absolutely cast iron, darling, and he doesn't like you to touch him either. I found all that rather sexy to begin with, but in the end I would have given anything just to have a cuddle and to feel some kind of physical connection. But he is great fun and if you get on he is awfully keen on the theatre and travel; we have had some truly super times together.'

'But not sex?'

'No, and on the occasions when we went away for the weekend or on holiday he always booked separate rooms. As I said, fun for a while, but in the end I needed more.'

We talked for quite a while and she gave me her name and address and said if I wanted to talk to her she was more than happy to chat over the phone or even meet up for coffee some time if I wanted to.

She was currently dating a much older Dom – a bear, she said – who, though he was less imaginative, liked nothing better than snuggling up in bed together at the end of a BDSM session. It was nice to talk to her. Like many of us who are involved in BDSM, I find that there is a limited number of people you can talk to about the life-style, so new friends who like to play are a plus. And so it was really on her say-so that I was heading across country to Gareth's farm, which was a couple of hours' drive away and situated in rolling hills outside a village that looked for all the world like something from a picture postcard.

I glanced down at the directions he had emailed me and then back out at the road. It had to be close. I was expect-ing a farmyard so almost drove past the gravelled entrance that was flanked by brick pillars and ornate gates.

Pulling into the driveway and following the tree-lined avenue down towards the house I began to realise that when Gareth had said 'farm' what he actually meant was 'small country estate'. I'd put a pair of wellington boots in the car as well as my high heels, just in case it was muddy, but there was really no need. This wasn't like any farm I had ever been to. I approached the front of the main house – an imposing Georgian pile – via a semi-circular gravel drive and parked by the steps that led up to the elegant front door. There was no one in sight.

The Georgian house was set among carefully manicured gardens and it was obvious, even at first glance, that you couldn't keep a place like this so well or so beautifully without staff, but if there was staff there didn't appear to be anyone around today. The whole place was quiet and still, with just the sounds of the birds and the wind in the trees. I felt a flutter of apprehension. I had told Gabbie where I was going, and sitting in the car I texted her to say that I had arrived. I'd barely sent the text before I got her reply. 'Have a good time. Let me know how it goes!'

I glanced up at the house. Gabbie thought I was going for lunch. I'd told her the address and that I was going to a farm and she had cooed over the idea of seeing sheep and dogs and assorted farm animals, and of Gareth being a rough-and-ready son of the soil. But it was quite obvious from the size and state of the place that I wasn't likely to be having a walk round the barns.

Gareth had emailed me my instructions for our meeting the day before and I had read them at least a dozen times before setting out. I had turned them over and over in my head during the drive over to his place. With my sense of anticipation and nervousness growing, I picked up my bag and shoes and headed for the house.

For anyone who thinks all this sounds totally mad, you are most probably right, but I had left all Gareth's details and where I was going on my desk top. Gabbie knew where I was and Gareth knew that I had told a friend of my whereabouts. I'd also spent hours talking to him on the phone prior to our meeting.

Now that I was actually at the house, I left my car close to the entrance with the door unlocked and the spare key tucked under the seat. I had spare clothes and an overcoat in the boot, just in case I had to make a fast get-away. Being a submissive doesn't mean that I'm a victim or a pushover and take whatever is doled out to me, nor do I assume that every Dom I meet is going to be trustworthy, and while I wanted to do what I was doing, by the same token I tried to be prepared in case things didn't turn out the way I planned.

So, there I was, excited, my pulse thumping in my ears as I crossed the driveway and climbed the steps. The front door was very lightly ajar, just like Gareth had said it would be. I stepped inside and, taking a long, calming breath, closed the door behind me.

Beyond the inner porch and another set of doors was a large, bright hallway with stairs rising up to a galleried landing. The house was gorgeous, decorated in comfortable country chic, though my main focus was not on the fixtures and fittings but on Gareth, who I could see waiting for me upstairs on the landing. He was watching my progress, but I had my instructions – I wasn't to acknowledge him, nor was I meant to look up or make eye contact.

A small painted wooden chair stood just inside the front door.

Gareth's emailed instructions were very clear. I was supposed to undress down to my underwear – a black satin basque, matching knickers and seamed black stockings – and leave my outdoor clothes and shoes folded neatly on the chair. I was then to put on the high heels, stand up straight, place my hands behind my back and wait for him to come down for me.

There was an edginess and excitement to this that cannot be explained or underestimated. I undressed slowly, slipping off my skirt and hanging it over the back rung of the chair, unbuttoning my blouse, slowly, slowly, aware that upstairs my every move was being watched by Gareth. There was an intensity that is hard to put into words and also, bizarrely, a sense of power.

I listened hard, wondering if I could pick out the sound of his breathing. I slipped the blouse off and hung it over the back of the chair, eased off my sensible shoes and slid into the impossibly high court shoes that I'd brought with me. Then slowly I put my hands behind my back and waited.

There was complete silence, total stillness. The waiting let me take stock, giving me a chance to gather my thoughts and also to calm down. I had been rushing around all morning, my brain racing, but now I was here, and I knew Gareth was here too. Time ticked by so very slowly. I let my breathing settle, felt my pulse slow. After a moment or two more, I heard his foot-steps on the stairs and felt a flicker of nervousness mingling with excitement.

'I'm so glad that you could make it, Sarah. I had wondered if you might back out at the last moment. And you've spoken to my friend about me?'

By 'friend' he meant his previous submissive.

'Yes, Sir,' I said, ensuring as per his instructions that I kept my eyes demurely lowered.

Gareth nodded. 'Good. I'm glad. She was a very good companion. A lovely woman.'

'Yes, Sir,' I said.

He was carrying a studded black leather collar and lead. 'Are you ready?' he asked.

I nodded.

'Come closer then,' he said, waving me towards him. 'Did you bring the contract with you?'

'Yes, Sir,' I said, and handed it to him.

He smiled. 'Good.'

It laid out in explicit detail what I would and wouldn't let Gareth do to me and what I expected him to do in return, which amounted to him keeping me safe, not abusing my trust and stopping if and when I wanted him to. Contracts are old-school BDSM and totally unenforceable, but it made me feel better to have the limits set down on paper, along with an agreed safe word.

Gareth scanned the sheets of paper and then signed them, tucking one signed copy into my handbag, which hung on the chair, and the other into his jacket pocket.

'And you're happy?' he asked.

I nodded.

Gareth smiled and very deftly fastened the collar around my neck before taking a moment to admire the effect. 'It suits you,' he said, looking me up and down. 'Next time, I want you to put your hair up,' he said, and with that he snapped on the lead and led me upstairs.

'In future I would like it if I could lead you on all fours,' he said, as we got to the first floor. 'There is no need for us to discuss it now but I would like you to consider it if we play again. For future reference, we will be using this room here,' he said, opening the door into a large, clinically white room, which was almost completely devoid of furniture except for a massage table standing in the centre of a bare wooden floor. There were mirrors all along the back wall, like those in a dance studio, a straight-backed chair, an armchair and various pulleys and ropes hanging from the ceiling. By the armchair was a flat trolley with drawers and various toys set out neatly on the top.

There was a row of colourful abstract prints hanging along the wall just inside the door, and beyond the pictures were two more doors. Gareth guided me further into the room.

'The first door', he said, as I looked around, 'is to a store cupboard for toys, clothes and props. I'll show you those another time. And this one here', he indicated the second door, 'is your bathroom, which you will use when you are with me. You will not go into any other areas of the house without my express permission. Is that clear?'

'Yes, Sir,' I said, looking past him into the bathroom, which was also completely white and had a rack piled with thick white towels and a robe hanging from a hook on one wall.

'I like my submissives to wear red lipstick while they are here and either have very short hair or to wear it up. The choice is yours. Do you understand?'

I nodded.

He frowned.

'Sorry, I meant yes, Sir.'

'That's better. You will find my preferred lipstick in the bathroom, along with perfume and something for your hair. While you are here you will leave the bathroom door open at all times, and when we are finished you may shower before you leave. Now, if you'd like to get ready.' He paused. 'Sometimes I will email you and just ask you to come up here and get ready for me. Is that acceptable?'

'Yes, Sir,' I said.

'Good. Now go and get ready, and don't be long. I will be waiting for you.'

Gareth sat down in the armchair while I headed to the bathroom.

The room was spotlessly clean and smelt of freesias, with an undertone of some sort of cleaner. There was a little tray on a glass shelf above the sink. On it was a new lip brush and a brand new and very expensive lipstick, along with a bottle of Chanel N°5, and in a little white bowl were all manner of hair accessories, scrunchies, grips and slides, all in black and all still in their wrappings.

I chose an oval clip from the bowl and, gathering my hair up, twisted it round and pinned it into place at the back of my head. I wasn't sure how long it would stay like that, but at least I had made the effort. The lipstick was as lush and thick as double cream and the colour made my skin look fabulous. As I glanced into the mirror to judge the overall effect I noticed that Gareth's chair was positioned so that he could watch me as I got ready.

There is something very powerful about transforming yourself into someone else's erotic fantasy, their object of desire. I couldn't help wondering who I was meant to be and when it was that Gareth had first decided that this was what constituted his perfect woman.

I checked my appearance; the lipstick and the change of hairstyle were enough to make my reflection seem unfamiliar. It was strangely liberating to pretend to be someone else. As Gareth watched me I added a quick spray of perfume, carefully blotted my lips on a tissue from a box on the vanity unit and dropped it into the bin before walking out to meet him, the main player in a fantasy not of my devising.

Gareth, still sitting in his armchair, nodded.

'Thank you,' he said. 'You look exquisite. Today we will take it slowly as it's our first time together. I prefer to tie my partners up, but I appreciate you may find that unsettling until we get to know each other better.' As he spoke Gareth got to his feet and indicated a length of rope that had been threaded through two rings which hung from the ceiling. 'So today I would like you to take hold of these and wind them around your wrists. Next time, if you feel comfortable with the idea, I would like to tie you to them. I usually use leather cuffs with sliding bolt catches.'

He held out a hand as if he was inviting me to dance or walk through an open door. As I stepped closer he handed me one end of the rope – a heavy woven hemp cord, taped and sewn at the ends – which I wrapped around my arm and held onto, and then he gave me the other end. The ends were suspended far enough apart so that by the time I had hold of each one I was stretched between them, arms akimbo, feet apart, but not uncomfortably so.

Once I was settled, Gareth smiled. 'Are you comfortable?'

I nodded. 'Yes, Sir.'

He moved slowly and deliberately, walking around me, running a hand over my shoulders and back, watching my face and my reaction, exploring my body and letting me settle, his movements and mine echoed in the wall of mirrors. He stood behind me, as if checking my appearance, then he bent down and pulled my knickers down, his face so close to me that I could feel his breath on my skin. He pulled them lower still so that I could step out of them.

'Next time,' he said, as he stood up, 'I want you to remove your pubic hair. I prefer my women completely naked. Do you understand?' He reached around me, his fingers teased the dark trimmed curls. 'All of this gone.'

'Yes, Sir,' I said, watching myself and him in the mirror. With Max, and with Alex in Whitby, I had spent a great deal of the time that we had played blindfolded, so it was extraordinary to be able to see what was going on, and watching it in a mirror gave it an oddly abstract, removed quality.

Gareth took a creamy-white ball gag from the trolley alongside his chair and held it out towards me as if he was offering me a treat. 'I would like you to wear this,' he said. 'Do you object?'

I shook my head. 'No, Sir,' I said.

'Good. Tell me if it is too tight. I want you to be comfortable.'

I opened my mouth so that he could put the hard rubber ball into my mouth; it tasted of chemicals, which made me think he had sterilised it.

'If you want me to stop at any time then just drop the ropes and I will stop immediately. Is that clear?'

I nodded as he fastened the gag into place, my painted lips smearing it with lipstick. He smiled at his handiwork before returning to the table and picking up a paddle. He flexed it. The paddle was maybe eighteen inches long, six wide, and made from some sort of flexible rubber. I'd never seen one quite like it before.

'I've found that this doesn't leave marks,' Gareth said conversationally, as he moved around me. He slipped a hand into the top of my basque, his fingers working over my flesh, lifting out first one breast and then the other, so that they sat above the cups of the basque.

Tucking the paddle under his arm, Gareth pulled a little tub of something out of the pocket of his trousers and, opening it, he dipped in a finger and then rubbed a little of the contents onto each of my nipples. His touch was firm and assured and made me shiver. Whatever was in the pot resembled rouge and coloured my skin to match my lips. It seemed that for him this was the final touch. He was arranging me to suit some inner vision of what or who it was that aroused him most and this, it seemed, was it.

He took up a position behind me. I watched him in the mirror, saw him close his eyes and take a moment or two to compose himself, and then watched, mesmerised, as he swung the paddle back. A split second later I felt it crack across my backside. I shrieked as I felt the pain. It was extraordinary to be able to watch what was happening and to see my body react to the sensation.

It was like being spanked, the impact hot and stinging, although the feeling was diffused across a wide area of skin. I bucked, pulling against the ropes; the sounds, my gasps and the thick guttural groan, muffled by the ball gag.

Before I could recover Gareth swung the paddle again, his face a mask of concentration. Only his eyes, bright with pleasure, gave away any clue as to what was going on inside his head. For me the sensations are a means to an end – strange as it may sound, I don't like pain, and I'm not impervious to it; things hurt me just as much as they hurt anyone else.

In real life I don't go around walking into doors or dropping things on my toe just for the buzz, but inside BDSM I do like the place pain takes me to and what it represents – a surrender, giving myself up to something I can't intellectualise away or entirely control. With BDSM the sensations are real, fierce and inescapable and bring me to myself, raw and whole and completely connected to my physical being, in a way that no other thing can.

Gareth drew back the paddle for another strike. The sensation rolled through me like a wave. And then there was another blow and another. The paddle made a distinctive slapping sound, and though the pain was far more bearable than the crop or a cane, it still hurt, making me writhe as each one hit home.

Between blows, I opened my eyes. I could see Gareth in the mirror, focused and glassy-eyed. He was as taut as a bow as he cracked the paddle, measuring the strength of the blows, his breathing ragged from the effort. The slaps were growing fiercer, getting a little harder, a little more painful with each stroke.

I strained against the ropes, biting down onto the ball gag, whimpering and moaning as each blow found its mark. I didn't count them. I drank them in. Although I was loath to admit it, Alex had reignited a need in me that I had been ignoring since I finished with Max. I needed this. I wanted it so very much. Gareth was fulfilling my fantasies as much as I was fulfilling his.

I cried out as the paddle found its mark yet again, finding myself tumbling headlong into the warm, almost trance-like stupor that the adrenaline-fuelled endorphin rush brought me. I could feel it bubbling through me. I felt drunk with it, and was absorbed not just by the sensation but by being able to watch myself in the mirror, the way my body moved and flexed, the way my face contorted, the way my hands clutched the ropes, and behind me Gareth, face set, leaning back into each blow. It was heady, heady stuff.

Finally Gareth set the paddle down on the trolley and unfastened the ball gag, helping me untangle the ropes from my arms, which were now red and indented with the pattern from the hemp where I had strained against it.

I was dizzy, intoxicated with the pain. Once I was untied, Gareth guided me over to the massage table and then bodily lifted me up onto it, giving me a glimpse of just how strong he was.

'Are you okay?' he asked.

'Yes, Sir,' I said. I was trembling.

'Do you want to stop? Have a break?'

I shook my head. I was fine and, in all honesty, hungry for whatever was coming next.

Gareth nodded. 'You have the safe word. If you want to stop all you have to do is ask.'

'Yes, Sir.'

His reminder and the fact that he was pulling on a pair of latex gloves made me reconsider my eagerness. We had discussed my limits and what I didn't want to do at some length, but I realised as Gareth opened a drawer in the trolley that I had no idea what he planned to do to me. I braced myself for whatever might follow, wondering if I might have to use the agreed safe word after all.

A study in concentration, Gareth took out a small bottle and poured a little puddle of baby oil into the palm of his hands. He stood up and came round to the top of the massage table and, taking the clip out of my hair, began to massage my head very, very slowly, working down over my neck and shoulders; it seemed that Gareth intended to explore every inch of my body – stroking, caressing, rubbing the oil into those parts of me that were exposed.

I realised, too, what his former submissive had meant about him not liking to be touched; it didn't just extend to me touching him, but him touching me. The fine latex gloves smoothed his path, making his caresses feel like liquid silk, but they were also a barrier, a way of ensuring that our flesh didn't touch.

I moaned softly as he worked his fingers into my muscles. It was one of the best massages I think I've ever had, and a stark contrast to the hot sting of the paddle.

'Sit up,' Gareth murmured. 'I want to undress you.'

I did as I was told and he undressed me, slowly, his fingers expertly undoing hooks and eyes on my corset, removing shoes and unrolling stockings, and arranging each item very carefully on the straight-backed chair alongside the massage bed.

Finally, totally naked, I lay back on the couch and he poured more oil onto his hands and the massage began again. Gareth worked on and on, his fingers exploring every last inch of me. He didn't speak or meet my eye but instead focused entirely on my body, working from the tips of my fingers down to the ends of my toes. It was beyond fabulous. I sighed and closed my eyes. He must have trained somewhere to be this good. I let myself sink back into the bed.

As I was sinking deeper and deeper into a near sleep-like state I felt a very subtle change in his touch and noticed that the way he was breathing had changed. I felt him catch hold of one of my breasts. My eyes snapped open. He took a clothes peg from the side table and closed it on my nipple. I gasped at the pain and the pressure. He grinned a lazy, contented grin and then took hold of my other breast, taking the nipple and stretching it away from my chest to apply the peg.

As our eyes met he asked me if I was still all right. I nodded, so blissed out, so relaxed that despite the pegs I could barely speak. Gareth smiled and picked up another peg, fixing it to the soft skin under my arm, one and then another and another and another. I was being pulled awake by the little bites and nips of the pegs' jaws. He picked up more and I closed my eyes, drinking in the tiny bites, the pegs picking out a pattern across my prone body, gradually sharpening my senses and dragging me back out of the relaxed state – and then I felt him stand up, felt him moving around the couch. He caught hold of my knees and opened my legs wide. I guessed what was coming and stiffened, my eyes snapping open.

He smiled down at me, opened my legs wider still and then, taking one of my labia between his thumb and forefinger, he opened the jaws of a peg wide and an instant later closed it on the soft, tender flesh. I gasped. The pressure was so intense and astonishing that it took my breath away and made me shriek, the pain radiating out in a dull throbbing arc from where the peg nipped.

Gareth stared at me, waiting, another peg already in his hand for the other side. The pain was dark and red; not a nip as I had anticipated so much as a steady aching pressure. As our eyes met he smiled. I knew that he could see the pain, but he could also see my need and hunger as clearly as I could see his. He was waiting for me to call a halt.

But I didn't. I didn't call the safe word, and so he clipped on the second peg and I bit my lip and whimpered, my eyes closed, my back arching, my breath coming in high, frantic gasps as the red-hot bite took hold.

'Good, good,' he murmured, stroking my thigh to settle me. 'Good, just breathe, gently, gently –'

And now, as my body started to accommodate the pain, I opened my eyes again. Gareth trickled baby oil down over the mound of my sex and worked it in. From the tray he took an object that looked for all the world like a miniature electric mixer, and as I watched he fitted a broad, bead-like head to it and then switched it on.

I jumped as it flicked into life, and he smiled.

It made a low, soft purring sound and I realised as he began to move it across my belly that it was a massage tool of some kind. Although it vibrated, its touch was smooth and almost frictionless as it glided over my skin in the warm oil.

Gareth brushed the massager across my inner thighs, letting it climb up my body. Despite the vibrations, the touch at its tip was as soft as a knowing tongue, the high rate of pulsations and the heady buzz adding to the intensity of the movement. Now he let it glide up towards my sex, stroking the outer lips first, making the pegs vibrate. I cried out as it made the pressure more intense, but before I could call a halt he moved the head of the little massager higher, finding the cleft in my sex, seeking out the bud of my clitoris.

I gasped as it found the spot, but this time it was with pure delight. I had occasionally used a vibrator in the past, but I didn't like them – the one I had, though, felt nothing like this. The action of the vibrating head was delicate and soft, the oscillation uneven and coming in intense and then softer bursts. Gareth – his expression unreadable – trickled more oil onto my body, lightly brushing the massager up and down, up and down, plucking pegs off my body with his other hand as he concentrated his attentions on my clitoris.

As I writhed and whimpered Gareth showed infinite patience and the ability to read my state of arousal, bringing me closer and closer to the edge only to snatch the prize away time and again, the sensations heightened by the little bites of pain from the teeth of the pegs. With each renewed pass over my clitoris I moved my body to meet the head of the massager, fighting the pain of the pegs, feeling the pleasure building inside me, getting closer and closer. His expression was calm and impassive, like a man conducting a complex experiment.

Finally, at the point when I couldn't take any more and I reached the peak, in the moment when I was feeling the intense rippling waves of orgasm, Gareth leaned in closer and plucked the pegs from my labia, one, two – and I screamed and thrashed from side to side, thunderstruck by the intensity, stunned at the mixture of pleasure and pain and the feeling of blood rushing back into the flesh. It was almost more than I could bear.

The combination was mind-blowing. Gasping for air, I felt as if I was falling and falling and falling – and when, moments later, I began to resurface and compose myself, and opened my eyes, I could see Gareth staring at me, watching me, as if taking in every last little detail of what he saw. Still breathing heavily, I ran my hands over my face and hair.

'Did you enjoy that?' he asked.

I nodded, still trembling, still shaken to the core. 'Yes, Sir,' I said.

'Not too much for you?'

'Almost,' I said, sitting up, the moment passing. 'The pegs hurt.'

'They were meant to. I'm very pleased you felt able to tolerate them, though. You could have asked me to stop.'

'I know,' I said. What I didn't add was that knowing I had a way out was, oddly enough, one of the things that made it possible to bear. I had the choice. I chose to experience the pain. I've given up trying to rationalise this stuff; I just accept now that this is what I enjoy, and I'm all the happier for accepting it as a given, rather than trying to justify or excuse it.

Gareth smiled, peeled off his gloves and dropped them into a little bin alongside the table before indicating that I should lie back down. I did as I was told and he covered me up with a soft fleece blanket from under the massage table.

'Just rest now. Give yourself a chance to recover,' he said. 'I will go and get us some tea. Or would you prefer coffee?'

'Tea would be lovely,' I said. I licked my lips. My mouth was dry. 'But what about you?' I added, painfully aware that I hadn't touched him at all – not so much as a peck on the cheek since I'd arrived, and I'd certainly not given him any kind of tangible sexual satisfaction.

Gareth smiled.

I felt cold now, and still in the aftermath of orgasm I started to shiver. Gareth tucked the blanket in around my shoulders.

'What about me?' he asked.

'You haven't come.' I couldn't think of any other way to put it.

Gareth nodded. 'You don't have to worry about me. I am very pleased with the way our first session together has gone, and believe me, I have all I need. I promise you. Now, you said tea?'

It was hard not to smile. Such a very civilised end to our session. I smiled.

'Yes, please,' I said.

'Good. Stay where you are. There is no need for you to move yet. You can have a shower once you've had your tea.'

He dimmed the lights before he went downstairs, leaving me curled up under the rug. I must have dozed off, because the next thing I knew I was being woken by Gareth stroking my hair off my face. It took me a few seconds to remember exactly where I was.

'You look so peaceful,' he said, as I yawned and rubbed my eyes. 'It seemed a shame to wake you really, but you should have something to drink.'

I shuffled myself up the couch, clutching the blanket to me, while Gareth adjusted the backrest so that I could sit comfortably. He handed me a glass of water to drink while he poured and served the tea in bone china cups. 'Milk or lemon?' he asked, setting the strainer down on a little matching bowl.

'Milk, please, Sir,' I said.

I noticed that my clothes from downstairs were now carefully folded over the straight-backed chair. For such a large man Gareth moved very quietly. I certainly hadn't heard him come back into the playroom while I was dozing.

'Would you like to come and visit me again?' he asked, offering me a plate of shortbread biscuits. Before I could answer Gareth held up a hand. 'Sorry. Forgive me. That was rude of me. You don't have to answer that now. I'll ring you or you may email me when you get home. I was talking to my previous submissive just before you arrived and she said that I should take it more slowly, give you time to consider how you feel about our arrangement, rather than rush you into making a decision about what comes next. Sorry.'

'You've talked about me?' I asked.

Gareth nodded. 'Yes, of course.' He sounded surprised that I might find that unusual. 'She and I still speak at least a couple of times a week. We used to get along very well. I still miss her. The good thing is that we have stayed close friends even though we're not seeing each other any more. She is seeing someone else now – I think she may have told you – so if you're worried about her, please let me reassure you that there is no chance we will be rekindling our relationship. She has made it perfectly clear that there is no way back.'

I smiled; it wasn't so much that Gareth was still talking to her, rather the fact that he had talked to her immediately before seeing me that I found slightly out of kilter.

'I am very fond of her,' Gareth continued. 'And I was sad to see her go, but I do also understand that she needed more, despite me making it perfectly clear from the outset that there is no more on offer.' As he spoke I was aware that Gareth was watching my face.

'And you think I'm going to be the same?' I said.

He nodded. 'Sadly, but if I got hung up on that I'd never meet anyone. Were you nervous about coming here today?'

'Yes.'

'How nervous?'

'Quite nervous.'

'Even though we had met and spoken on the phone?'

I nodded. 'I'd be foolish if I wasn't a bit nervous.' I laughed. 'Here I am, stark naked in a stranger's house; why would I not be nervous? The thing is, if I want this life-style then there is always going to be a risk, isn't there?'

Gareth nodded. 'That is true for both of us.'

I glanced at him. That hadn't really occurred to me before.

'From the Dom's point of view, we're taking a consider-able risk too. Society would see me as the aggressor, not the victim, if anything went wrong while you were here.' He took a sip of tea. 'So we both have to be careful. There are many shades of mad and damaged around, on both sides of the equation. So I trust my previous sub's judgement when it comes to helping me find someone to play with.'

'You get your ex-sub to vet your women for you?' I asked.

Gareth smiled. 'It's not entirely on her say-so but yes, to some degree, and why not? She says she is happy to do it. Can you think of a better idea?'

'It seems a bit perverse,' I said.

Gareth threw back his head and roared with laughter. 'Perverse? Really?' he said. 'And this isn't?' He lifted his hands to encompass the playroom, with its ropes, pegs and paddles.

'Okay, I see your point. Given what we're doing, maybe it's not that perverse, but it still seems a pretty odd thing to do.'

'I know, but she's been a good friend and I really do value her opinion. I'm not great at reading other people's motives. I think that may well be a male thing, but I know from experience that I'm worse than most. So I ask my ex.'

He grinned. 'Alternatively I just bring a woman home, I tie her up and beat her. She could report me for assault or worse, and let's face it, anyone coming in here earlier would be dragging me off in handcuffs, not you. The risk is shared, but from the outside looking in, if anyone found us, then the fault, the risk, would be mine. So I want to try to ensure that the women I play with are not just submissive but also stable and sane. It's not always easy. There are a lot of wannabees and fantasists out there. No one wants some lunatic rushing to the tabloids or the police, screaming blue murder and claiming I'm some sort of sadistic pervert.' His grin widened. 'Even if I am. Which is why I let my ex talk to them first.' He refilled his teacup.

I nodded. It made sense. Sort of.

'I'm pleased I passed,' I said, taking another biscuit.

'She told me that she thought you sounded nice, with a warm personality, and grounded.'

I laughed. It made me sound like the ideal candidate for a job as a doctor's receptionist. 'And how about you, what do you think?'

'My opinion is that you and I will get along very well for the time being, but I suspect that you, too, will be wanting more than I have to offer before long. Now, if you'd like to have a shower and get dressed then please, feel free. There is a robe and towels in the shower room.'

As I stood under the torrent of hot water and rinsed away the baby oil, the perfume and the last of the red lipstick, I had time to reflect on what Gareth had said. He was right. I'd never really considered just how thin a line Doms walked in their search to find the right woman, nor how vulnerable a position they put themselves in. Even the idea of the contract made more sense after talking to him.

Something else that struck me as I lathered my hair was that, despite crying off getting involved with Alex, I did need to feel more of an emotional connection with my Dom for the play to have any real significance. Today had felt good and was certainly satisfying if the yardstick was purely about orgasm and physical satisfaction, but Gareth was right: what he offered wasn't something I wanted for the long term. It felt like eating chocolate when what you really wanted was a proper meal. I needed a relationship to have the space to grow and develop over time. In the end, what it boiled down to was that I needed to be loved, and I knew – sex or no sex – that that wasn't on offer with Gareth. So he was absolutely right when he said that this arrangement would do me for a while, but it wasn't what I was really looking for.

When I had showered, dried and dressed, Gareth, who was waiting for me outside the bathroom, guided me back downstairs and showed me out to my car. As we got to the door he handed me a little bunch of flowers that looked as if they had been picked from the garden, their stems all tied up with raffia. They were beautiful and it was a lovely gesture.

'Drive safely and please text me to let me know that you have arrived home. I'll phone you in the week,' he said, opening the car door for me. As he said goodbye, Gareth made no move to hug or kiss me or even shake my hand, and nothing about his body language encouraged me to give any of those things a try.

I drove home wondering what it was I actually wanted from a BDSM relationship. When I got home I sent Gareth a 'Thank you for a lovely afternoon' email and popped the flowers into a little vase on my desk.

That evening Alex rang. I had thought there was a chance that I might hear from Gareth too, but there was nothing, not so much as a text. Obviously his ex-sub hadn't explained to him that women, even women who are neither needy nor mad, like a little acknowledgement of an intimate moment shared.

'So,' Alex said, when I picked up the phone, 'how did today's audition for the perfect Dom go?'

'Okay,' I replied.

I'd been working on the new book since I got home from seeing Gareth. Alex's call had broken my concentration and looking up at the clock made me realise that it was high time I called it a day. With the phone gripped between my chin and shoulder I switched off the computer and headed out to the kitchen, chatting to Alex as I went. It was good to hear his voice.

'So, you're not that impressed then?' he said.

'I didn't say that.' I propped the phone up on top of the breadbin while I poured myself a glass of wine.

'You didn't have to say anything, I can hear it in your voice.'

'Don't jump to conclusions, Alex. However it went, I'm not going to give you a blow-by-blow account of my afternoon, okay?'

'When you say blow-by-blow ...' Alex said jokily, leaving the sentence unfinished and hanging between us so that the snippet of silence filled with all manner of sexual innuendo.

I laughed. 'Stop it! I'm not telling you about it, or do you get off on that kind of thing?'

'Hardly, not when I would like it to be me,' he said. 'I just wanted to be certain that you were okay and that he wasn't a patch on me.'

I didn't intend to pander to his ego. I carried the phone into the sitting room and put a match to the log fire that I had laid before I went out. My dog padded out of his basket in the office to take his place on the hearthrug.

'So, you're calling *because* ...?'

'Because I wanted to see how you were, make sure you were okay. And to ask if you'd like to come to a do with me.'

'A *do*?'

'Uh-huh, an event, a night out, a big flashy dinner with dancing and an old-style dance band and gallons of champagne. It's a promotional event for a company I'm doing some work with at the moment, and they sent me a plus one.'

'And you haven't got anyone else who'll go with you?' I joked.

'Oh, you can be so cruel,' Alex said, pretending to wince. 'Actually I was inviting you because I enjoy your company and I'd really like to see you again.'

'And the six months rule?'

'We never said we wouldn't go out during that time, did we? I didn't think that was part of the deal?'

'No, but –'

'And it doesn't sound to me like this afternoon was the start of any kind of happy ever after, so say yes. Go on, you know you want to.'

He was right, I did.

'No strings,' he said. 'Just ropes and maybe a pair of handcuffs. Oh, and a blindfold.'

I laughed.

'When is this *do*?'

'In a couple of months' time. I just wanted to make sure you weren't double booked. I could come and pick you up and we could stay over. It's black tie, lots of posh frocks. Actually, maybe we could go out and get you something really special to wear. I've always fancied being a sugar daddy, sitting outside the changing room in some plush frock shop while assistants run around and some pretty little thing tries on outfits for my approval.'

I laughed. 'Alex, it's a great fantasy but there is no way I'd pass for a pretty little thing in anyone's books.'

'Don't sell yourself short; you could very easily be my pretty little thing,' he teased. One thing about Alex was that he made me smile. 'How about we have a day's shopping and I could buy you an outfit, dress you exactly how I wanted and –'

'Stop,' I laughed.

'Oh come on, come and play with me. I've missed you. We could make a proper day of it. A nice long lazy lunch, shopping … I know the perfect place. Just say yes.'

Who could resist?

Me.

'No,' I said.

'No? Oh, come off it, it'll be fun, and tell me a woman who can resist the promise of shopping and food? I've got visions of us locked in a changing room in some high-end department store, you in black stockings and suspenders, your back up against the wall of the cubicle, legs round my waist, and me –'

I like a man with an imagination.

'Have you been in any women's changing rooms lately?' I asked, cutting him off in mid-flow. 'The walls are about as thick as cardboard and the doors start at knee height in most of them.'

'Adds to the excitement,' said Alex.

'And the chances of getting arrested.'

'Spoilsport. So are you going to say yes?'

'To what?'

'Shopping and a night out on the town dancing under the stars to the strains of a big band?'

I hesitated long enough for Alex to say: 'Good, that's decided. I'll email you the details of the do and we can sort out the shopping trip. I need a new bow tie.'

I sighed. 'I'll check my diary.'

'Did I browbeat you?'

'Not really. It's just been a long day.'

His tone changed. 'You want to talk about it?'

'No, not really, and particularly not to you. You're part of the problem, not the solution.'

'I could come over.'

'And that would make it better? You live miles away.'

'Not that far, and you're worth it. I could bring us a bottle of wine and snuggle up to you all night long.'

In that moment, I realised I was sorely tempted to cave in. I could do with a cuddle – hardly the heights of erotic BDSM fun, but highly appealing.

For those on the outside looking in, it's important to point out that Dom-sub relationships aren't just about pain. They can be about control and power, but they can also be about giving you what you need, a feeling of security, comfort, approval; the closest we get as adults to unconditional love.

But hadn't I already told Alex that I was reluctant to accept what he had to offer? Wasn't that as much because I didn't want to lead him on or hurt him as for my own sake?

'Thank you, it's a lovely thought, but I think I'm going to have some supper, watch rubbish on the TV and then go to bed.'

'Okay, but if you need me –' he left the offer hanging.

'Actually, I do,' I said, catching sight of Joan's invitation tucked behind a candlestick on the mantelpiece. 'Do you fancy coming to a wedding with me?'

'Is there a four-poster bed involved?'

I laughed. 'No, not this time. Does that mean you won't come?'

'No, I was just checking so I know what to pack.'

'It's one of my best friends. Joan.'

'One of the gang of four,' said Alex.

'That's right.'

'I remember you telling me, and in that case I would be honoured. When is it?'

I opened the envelope and slipped out the card and told him the date.

'I'll put it in my diary. And you're sure you want to take me and not today's Dom?'

'Absolutely certain,' I said.

# Chapter Nine

I went to visit Gareth once or twice more before I decided categorically that he had been right about me. And when it came down to it, I had been right about me too. I needed a lot more than just the physical side of BDSM, and despite Gareth being a technical whiz kid when it came to tying women up, tying them down and bringing them to earth-shattering, teeth-chattering, feels-like-you've-been-electrocuted orgasm, he had been completely candid from the outset when he said that he was looking for nothing beyond the structured, rigid framework of simple BDSM encounters and had nothing more to offer.

In some ways I was quite envious that what he wanted and could get were so very clearly defined, and when we talked, when we weren't playing, it was obvious that Gareth was very happy with the arrangement. He said that he hoped one day to find someone to play with long term, someone who would be content with his terms of engagement. He was a cultured and intelligent man and would have liked someone who wanted to travel with him, go to the theatre and the opera, but who nonetheless could remain at a rather chilly distance. I knew it wasn't for me. I needed something altogether warmer and less clinical.

I had thought that perhaps his no-strings approach would be a good way for me to have my needs met while I worked out exactly what it was I wanted and that I could cope with it, but on a second outing I knew it would just make me unhappy and in some way devalue the experience if it was reduced to a purely physical function.

Gareth and I parted on good terms. He said if I ever wanted to come back and spend the afternoon in his playroom he would be more than happy to oblige. All I had to do was ring or email him. As we said our goodbyes I was slightly concerned that he might ask me to join his vetting panel for future submissives, but fortunately Gareth was too busy cutting me some flowers from his precious and very beautiful garden to ask.

I met up for brunch with Alfie. Alfie was a man who, among many other things, liked to write obscenities on his submissives and then take them out for the evening. The words and phrases, which he very carefully composed, were covered by just a fraction of an inch of fabric, written just below a plunging neck line or above the hemline of a skirt. His expectation and desire grew as he imagined the words, warm and waiting for him to re-read them, on the naked skin of the women he was escorting.

Alfie told me he liked to read his subs the way he read books when he first learned to read at school, running his fingers under each word in turn and saying them aloud. He was tall and slim and nice-looking in an earnest, studious way. He explained that he didn't just write obscenities; sometimes he preferred poetry or a phrase or descriptive passage that excited him from a novel. Sometimes his play partner would bring along a piece of text that she liked and he would write it on her while she dictated.

Alfie said: 'The idea of the human body as a blank canvas is something that really turns me on,' and then he paused and smiled. 'I think you either get it or you don't. No halfway measures.'

Over a huge plate of ham and eggs we talked about how it made him feel, writing on human flesh, the way skin puckered up under the tip of the felt tip and how the ink sometimes spread and flowed in unexpected ways. He told me about how movement would erase or soften the letters at points on the body as his subbie walked or sat. He said that he had always wished that he could draw. Alfie would like to draw on his women.

When I suggested that perhaps he ought to take up tattooing he said that didn't appeal to him at all. He preferred the fleeting and changeable possibilities of felt-tip pens, and the chance to add a new phrase, word or poem to reflect his mood whenever his chose.

We discussed marker pens. He talked about which ones stayed on the body and remained legible, the words crisp and clear, but would also wash off easily without permanently marking the submissive's clothing or staining the skin, and which were to be avoided as they were all but bombproof and couldn't be washed or even scrubbed off, but instead took days to fade and even then left a mark that would only vanish over time.

He told me about a fantasy he had, about hiring a Greek villa for a couple of weeks, somewhere that was isolated, with its own beach and a pool, so that he and his sub could have the time and the privacy for him to write all over her and then just let the words fade as she swam and bathed in the sunshine.

He told me about a couple he had met through the website we were both on; the husband had brought his wife to Alfie's house for a BDSM session and during the whole thing had just sat in a chair and watched while the wife told my brunch date her dirtiest, rawest and raunchiest innermost thoughts, from which Alfie and the husband had chosen pertinent words and phrases and then written them on the wife's body.

Apparently the two of them – the husband and wife – had been delighted with the result and at having a fantasy they had imagined finally come to fruition. She left fully dressed with the words still on her, covered by her clothes. Alfie said the pair could barely keep their hands off each other.

As we sat there, me mopping up the last of the juices on my plate with a hash brown, Alfie looked longingly at my hand and arm where it vanished into the sleeve of my cardigan.

'I could write something for you, if you like,' he said, gently stroking a finger over the bump of my wrist bone where it joined my hand. 'On your arm. I've brought a pen with me. Just one word. You could see how it feels.'

I smiled, trying to think of a polite way to decline. Not that Alfie was creepy or unpleasant or pushy in any way, far from it. He appeared nothing other than normal and was quite good-looking in rangy way. He was in his late thirties, well dressed, intelligent, articulate and good company. In lots of ways he would make an ideal Dom for someone, and was certainly the ideal brunch date – but it just wasn't my thing.

The bottom line is you're looking for someone with matching or complementary kinks, or someone who is prepared to try what you have to offer or at the very least is attracted to it. I didn't think being a human notice board was my thing and didn't fancy Alfie enough to want to give it a try. But that didn't mean I wasn't curious.

'What would you write?' I asked.

He thought for a moment. 'For a first time? Probably something overtly sexual,' he said thoughtfully. 'Something coarse, something memorable, so that when you got home you would look at it and it would have a real impact. There is a shock value in seeing words on your body. "Slut" or "whore",' he said. 'It would need to be something strong. I could write it in reverse, if you like, so that you could read it in the mirror.'

I smiled and poured myself another cup of tea.

Once you scratch the surface, people's fantasies and their sexual preferences are incredibly varied and diverse, and very few people I met on my journey could in any way be described at outwardly weird or different, and certainly not freaks or monsters. I find other people's fetishes and desires endlessly fascinating, and it is always an extraordinary privilege to discover what goes on in another person's head.

It was a different matter when it came to the reality of playing out a BDSM scene with them. I reserve the right to be as prudish, judgemental or perverse as the next person. Trust me, being into BDSM does not necessarily make you broadminded. To put it another way, one man's kink is another man's 'no way, are you barking mad?'

Alfie took my silence as potential agreement and brought a selection of felt-tips out of his jacket pocket. 'So, what do you think?' he said, eyes bright, fanning them out across the table top so that presumably I could pick a colour.

My smile held. 'Thank you, but no thank you. I don't think it's really my thing,' I said.

He nodded, totally unfazed. 'Fair enough, although maybe you should try it?' he suggested. 'You've got the most beautiful skin. You might like it.'

'I don't think so.'

'Okay.' He looked genuinely disappointed. 'It's been good to meet you. I hope you find what you're looking for,' he said, slipping the pens back into his pocket.

'You too,' I said.

We kissed each other on the cheek and hugged.

As he paid the bill the cuff of his shirt rode up just fraction and I thought I caught a glimpse of two words, written in black in among the hair on his arm. I can't be certain, but I think it said: 'Good Boy.'

I had coffee with another guy who seemed to think I would get a sexual charge from doing his cleaning, and a lovely man who liked to keep his visiting subs in a large dog cage in his kitchen by the Aga, preferably naked or dressed in an outfit of his choosing. It was, he said, only for a couple of hours at a time while he ate his supper and watched the news, and I wouldn't be bored as there were lots of blankets and toys in there.

'Toys?' I asked casually, aware that I was walking into a part of the BDSM world I knew almost nothing about.

'Yes, you know, rubber balls, bones, squeaky things, chewy sticks,' he said. 'The kinds of things that dogs like.'

'Really,' I said, nodding politely.

People take their fetishes very seriously and one man's meat is another man's lady-sized Dalmatian. He told me that he liked to hand-feed titbits to his pet through the bars, and then he showed me some pictures on his phone of his previous girlfriend, her face pixelated out.

I reminded myself again as I looked at the images that whoever I played with had to agree to a cast-iron no-photos, no-video clause. I had no desire to have any of my finer features shared on someone's iPhone for the edification of the next in line.

The woman in the photo was blonde, shapely and obviously worked out. (Another reason why I didn't want to be in photos: for me, sexy is as much if not more about what's going on in your head as your body.)

His previous partner was wearing long floppy ears, had spots and whiskers drawn on and was wearing a ball gag which incorporated something that looked like a dog's nose.

I hadn't come across anyone who had taken a human pet fetish this far before, so, ever curious, I asked him how he'd got into it. He explained that his previous girlfriend, the lady Dalmatian, had introduced him to it and it had just clicked. She and I were around the same age, so while I had been dreaming of being tied up she had been imagining rolling over to have her tummy tickled and fetching sticks. Takes all sorts.

'Did you meet her on a fetish website?' I asked conversationally, flicking through the images, which I have to say were totally fascinating. In one she was begging, hands up like paws, her dog name picked out in rhinestones on an oversized nametag.

'Oh no,' he said. 'I have gone on a couple of websites since we split up, because it's a bit of a niche thing really, especially if you factor in the Ds thing, and I've met some lovely people. But no, we met in the pet-food aisle of our local supermarket. She was buying dog treats and we just got talking, and one thing led to another.'

I kept my eyes firmly fixed on the images on the phone. I can't imagine the conversation that led from buying a packet of rawhide chewies to getting a woman naked in a dog cage wearing a butt plug with a tail attached, but I was prepared to take his word for it. Since they had split up, which he was quick to point out were for reasons totally unrelated to the dog fetish, he had come across several subs who wanted to be pets – dogs, cats, horses (pony girls have lots of dedicated websites) and even one who wanted to be a rabbit – but none of them had clicked with him.

He was pleased to meet me, but he said he could see that it wasn't really my kind of thing, though if I ever changed my mind we could take it one step at a time, work up slowly, maybe start with a collar and the ears. I thanked him for sharing his fantasy with me. It was fascinating, but he was right, it wasn't what I was looking for. Back to the drawing board.

When I got home Alex had rung to remind me about the company party and our planned day out shopping.

'Oh, yes, that looks fabulous. Can you just turn round again, Sarah, so that we can take a look at the back? I love that. Don't you?' said Alex, to the female assistant in the dress shop.

We'd been in the shop for the best part of an hour, maybe longer … It felt like longer. A. Lot. Longer.

The woman who was serving us nodded and tweaked something on the bodice, tugging the dress into shape.

'Yes, I think this is definitely the one,' the woman said triumphantly. 'Let me just help you on with the jacket, shall I?' She slipped it off the hanger and held it up while I put it on. 'There we are. See, now that looks lovely. You'll have to do something with your hair, obviously,' said the woman, casting a critical eye over the whole ensemble. Although she appeared to be talking to me, a lot of her remarks were aimed at Alex, who nodded sagely.

'She could wear it up, maybe,' suggested Alex, as the woman pulled at the bottom of the jacket so that it sat squarely across my shoulders.

She nodded in agreement and then ran her hands back over my hair. 'Or even just back off her face,' she said. 'We've got some lovely combs in the shop. Or maybe you could take it all over to one side and have a clip.'

I was standing just outside the changing room in the back of an old-fashioned ladies' dress shop being styled by the two of them, who had struck up an almost instant rapport.

The two of them were talking about me as if I wasn't there. Not that I minded in this particular case because between them they were doing a great job of giving me a fashion makeover. I loved the clothes they'd picked out, although I wouldn't have chosen them myself. Between them they were deciding what I should wear to Alex's black-tie dinner.

He and the assistant – who I suspected might also be the shop owner and was the wrong side of sixty, exquisitely dressed, coiffured and made up – made a formidable team.

When we'd gone inside, I had said something along the lines of: 'I'm really not sure what I'm looking for.' Once the woman realised that Alex was serious about buying me something fabulous and we weren't just time-wasting window shoppers, she took this as a personal challenge.

Alex had explained to her where we were going. She looked impressed and looked me up and down before running a knowing eye and finger along the shop rail, picking out half a dozen dresses, along with shoes and a couple of wraps to finish off the look.

Alex, meanwhile, was living out part of his fantasy. There was a pair of leather tub chairs in the back room, set either side of a small table that had newspapers and magazines on it and was obviously meant for husbands, lovers, partners and friends. He was currently sitting in one drinking a cup of coffee that the Saturday girl had made for him, while the senior assistant zipped me into one evening dress after another.

It had been a long time since I'd thought about formal evening dresses. The woman had already decided that cocktail length was out and that I had to go for the full-length classic number. Alex agreed, and this, it seemed, was it: a sea-greeny-blue dress with a little boxy jacket. Although it looked quite soft, it was structured, beautifully cut and lightly boned so that it made the most of my curves. It also cost more than I'd spent on clothes in the last six months – not that Alex seemed perturbed by the price tag.

Now that the look was complete the woman walked around me and took a long, hard, appraising look. 'It's lovely, and the colour is perfect. Can you just slip the jacket back off for me?'

I did as I was told.

She moved in closer. 'I think we should take the hem up a little bit, and just take a tad out of here.' Expertly she pulled up the straps at the back, which lifted my breasts up.

Alex nodded his approval. His expression was mischievous. 'Perfect,' he said.

'And then if we just take a little out of here to give the whole thing a bit of oomph ...' The woman pinched in a little pleat of fabric on the sides.

Alex's gaze caught mine. 'In my opinion you can never have too much oomph,' he said. Was it possible that choosing an evening dress can make you feel horny? Apparently it was. He grinned and took a sip from his cup, eyes alight over the rim.

The woman, meanwhile, strapped a little band with a pin cushion on it to her wrist and began to make the necessary adjustments, pulling the fabric in here and there, making a little tuck in the back, getting me to stand on a box while she adjusted the hem – every move watched by Alex. By the time she was done and I had put the jacket back on, the dress looked even more fabulous. She stood back to admire her handiwork. Alex stood back to admire me and then applauded.

'Bravo, *bellissimo*! That is amazing, you're a genius,' he said. The woman blushed and giggled like a teenager.

While I looked at myself in the mirror, they discussed how long it would take to make the alterations, whether I should take the shoes as well (I did) and what if any jewellery I needed. Finally they debated whether I needed to come back to try the dress on when Alex picked it up. The consensus was that, yes, I did, which I guessed from Alex's expression played right into his hands.

Which was when the shop bell rang. The woman peeked around the doorway of the back room into the shop. I could see from her expression that she was torn between wanting to stay and help us and going out to attend to whoever had just walked into the shop. After all, the hard work of choosing and pinning was done, and the decisions were made.

'Do you want to go and serve?' I asked, as she turned her attention back to Alex and me. She looked slightly nonplussed, not wanting to be impolite and presumably feeling obliged to see this sale through to the bitter end.

'It's fine,' she said. 'I'm sure Melanie can cope ...' She may have said it, but we all knew she didn't mean it.

'I don't mind, really.' I said. After all, I was busy admiring my reflection in the full-length mirror and trying to ignore the look on Alex's face.

'Are you sure you wouldn't mind? I just need to go and have a quick word –' the woman said, glancing back towards the shop.

'No, not at all,' Alex said, waving her away before I could reply. 'Take your time. We're fine. Really.'

I shot him a look; he shrugged.

'Will you be able to take the dress off?' she asked solicitously.

Alex got to his feet. 'Oh, I think so,' he said. 'I can help, can't I, Sarah?'

I managed to keep a straight face. The instant the woman had vanished back into the shop Alex was on his feet and whipped back the heavy velvet curtain that divided the changing area from the rest of the room.

'Shall we?' he said, holding it to one side and waving me in.

I raised my eyebrows.

'Notice', he said, indicating the curtain, 'that it reaches right down to the floor and then some.'

I nodded and stepped past him. There was a full-length mirror on one wall and a fancy painted chair standing up against the partition wall. All the way along the back wall was a pink velvet-covered shelf seat. My clothes were on the shelf.

The very instant the curtain dropped back to the floor Alex grabbed me and kissed me hard. I felt my whole body responding to his and I kissed him back with equal fervour. His lips were hard and insistent and despite my intentions of playing it cool, I wanted him. I wanted him a lot. Alex fumbled my fabulous jacket off and let it drop to the floor.

'Hang on, hang on,' I said breathlessly, pushing him away as he started on the dress. 'It's all pinned together.'

'I don't care,' he growled.

'Well I do! I don't want them sticking in me or her having to do them again.'

'Who is the Master here?' he said, eyes dark with desire and that twist of mischief that he had about him. 'Here, let me.'

He turned me around and started to unfasten the zip, carefully at first, then ripping it down, sliding his hands in around my waist easing me out of the silky sheath. I shivered at his touch. He leaned in closer and kissed my neck, tracking kisses over the sensitive flesh, pressing his lips to the spot where my ear met my neck, his tongue lapping, lips planting a flurry of kisses.

I closed my eyes, drinking in the sensations. Alex's hands circled around to my front, cupping my breasts, squeezing them tightly – so tightly that I gasped.

'God, that feels so good,' he murmured, catching my hard nipples between his thumbs and forefingers, rolling and tugging at them. I could feel his excitement building, mirroring my own. This was madness.

I groaned as his kisses grew more and more intense. The dress, my fabulous, fabulous dress, was all but forgotten and fell to the floor around my feet. Alex pushed me forward so that my hands were flat against the dividing wall of the changing room and ran his hands down over my waist, over my hips and under the sides of my knickers and pulled them down.

'God, you look amazing. Just stay like that, stay there,' he said. 'I've been thinking about this since we came in here. I'm going to fuck you. You know that, don't you?'

I groaned. This was totally, totally crazy. His hand fell away and I heard his zip unfasten, followed by the sound of him ripping open a condom wrapper, and then I felt the hard insistent press of his cock as it brushed the insides of my thighs, seeking entry, engorged and unstoppable.

I bent lower so that I was at a better angle, tipping my pelvis to let him in. Then I reached between my legs to guide Alex inside me and this time is was he who groaned. I could feel my body opening as he slid home; I was wet and hungry and as eager as he was. It *was* madness, total madness, and I didn't care.

I wondered how long we had. A minute, maybe two before the woman came back. What if she opened the curtains?

His cock filled me, making me gasp, and then he took hold of my hips and pulled me back hard onto him. I closed my eyes as we fell into a rhythm and tried hard not to make a sound, not to cry out, not to moan with pleasure. We couldn't be long, we couldn't be long – my mind was racing, trying to hang onto sensible thoughts, namely that we shouldn't be doing this at all.

Alex tangled his fingers in my hair and pulled my head back. I stifled a cry and he leaned in and bit my shoulder. As he pushed deeper still I slipped my hand between my legs. I was so aroused, so very, very turned on that the slightest touch lit great sparks of light behind my eyes. Alex moved in and out of me, breathing hard, pulling me onto his shaft. I moved with him, my fingers working, stroking his balls, stroking my clitoris, exploring the warm, wet place where our bodies joined.

I glanced across at our reflection in the changing-room mirror. Please, God, let no one walk in and catch us, I thought. I looked like some wild animal rutting and Alex little better, hunched over me, his face a picture of concentration as he drove into me again and again.

Somewhere out on the periphery of my hearing I could pick out the shop assistant talking to her new customer, hear light chatter amid female laugher; but here, in here, in this tiny closeted space, all there was was sex and Alex and me, and a roaring hunger that refused to be ignored.

I knew that we didn't have long before the shop assistant came back. The prospect of getting caught – the embarrassment, the shame – added a real frisson and an urgency that drove us both on. I guessed that under the circumstances Alex was hardly likely to string it out. I could already sense that he was close to the edge and he wasn't alone. As I matched Alex stroke for stroke my fingers were joined by his. His touch was firm and knowing. It was enough. The touch of his fingertips caressing my clitoris was enough to send me tumbling over the edge in a great rolling sea of orgasm. I was amazed that it was happening so quickly. The pleasure spread through me, making me go weak at the knees. Alex held me close as I gasped, my sex tightening around him, sucking him dry, pulling him deeper.

When he realised that I was coming I heard the breath catch in Alex's throat, and like a house of cards he came tumbling down after me, gasping, struggling for breath, as his thrusts grew more and more ragged and instinctive.

His fingers tightened around my hip bones and dragged me back onto him, milking every last sensation, every shred of pleasure. Then I felt him shudder, felt his cock pulse deep inside me, and he came long and hard, with a deep animalistic sigh of release.

When it was over we stood for a few seconds, hot, breathless, panting, hunched over in among the wreckage of the evening dress and my clothes, both spent, both shaking and trying very hard to keep upright and quiet. Looking up I could see his face in the mirror. He was grinning.

After slowly sliding out of me Alex dealt with the condom, while I made an effort to compose myself. I glanced in the mirror. My hair was all over the place; I needed a hairbrush and to wipe the cat-that-got-the-cream smile off my face. I pulled up my knickers and stepped out of the crumpled folds of the evening dress, scanning the floor and the shelf. My handbag had to be around somewhere. Alex pulled up his trousers, tucked in his shirt and zipped up his flies, taking a moment or two to catch his breath.

'You're crazy,' I said.

'And you're not?' he murmured, grabbing hold of my hair and kissing me hard.

'Everything all right in there?' asked the shop assistant from outside the curtain.

'Just fine,' said Alex, in a completely normal cheery voice. 'It was a bit of a job but we got there in the end.'

He was right about that.

'Do you need a hand?' asked the woman.

Alex looked at me and raised his eyebrows.

'No, we're fine,' I said hastily.

'Just be careful with the pins,' she called through the closed curtain. 'If you could try to leave them in … But you don't want to get pricked, do you?'

Our eyes met. There was no real answer to that.

'Won't be a second,' I said, breaking eye contact with Alex and finally spotting my handbag, which was under the jacket I had dropped on the floor with the evening dress.

As I retrieved it Alex ran his fingers back through his hair, picked up the evening dress and very carefully hung it over his arm and smoothed it out. Taking the jacket from me he slipped out around the curtain, leaving me to compose myself. It was going to take a while. I took a deep breath and a long, hard look in the mirror. My eyes were bright, my skin flushed and glowing. I was really hoping the lady in the shop might take my post-coital blush for excitement. I raked the hairbrush through my hair, making an effort to get my act together and get dressed. I found the bra I'd taken off to try the dress on. I pulled on my jeans and boots and buttoned my shirt. Rooting through my handbag I tracked down my lipstick and did a quick touch-up job. The overall effect wasn't too bad.

When I was ready I took one last look around. It seemed odd that the changing room looked so tidy, with no physical trace of what had gone on moments earlier. As I was about to open the curtain it occurred to me that there might be one last thing I hadn't accounted for. I took the tiny perfume bottle I had in my make-up bag and gave the place a quick spray to mask any lingering scent of sex. I whisked open the curtain, pulling it all the way open so that the air could clear.

There was no one in the back room but out in the shop Alex and the shop assistant were waiting for me. They were both smiling.

'We've just been discussing when you're going to come back to pick up your outfit,' said the woman, who had one eye on the other assistant who was busy rehanging the dress and putting a label on it. 'We've got the new season's stock arriving in a couple of weeks. Maybe you'd like to join our mailing list? We have an opening evening – canapés, wine …'

She handed me a card. I glanced at Alex, who waved me into action. 'Yes, why not,' he said. 'Fill it in.'

'He's keen. He can't wait to come back and do it again,' laughed the woman.

I raised my eyebrows and looked at Alex, who just smiled and said: 'We've had a fabulous time, haven't we, Sarah? I said to the lady here we can't wait to come again.'

I didn't trust myself to speak.

# Chapter Ten

Back on my search for Master Right, the next Dom on my list was called Charles and he invited me to have afternoon tea with him at a local beauty spot, which was famous for its tearoom and home-baked cakes. Who could refuse? He emailed me the directions for how to get there, along with a set of instructions:

Sarah, tomorrow when we meet do not wear make-up, antiperspirant, body lotion or perfume. I prefer my women close to how nature intended them. As a Master I have strict regulations and rules regarding my submissives and their appearance. I prefer long hair and will expect you to grow yours if you prove to be a suitable candidate. I like my women to be proud of their femininity. When in public and in my company I expect my submissives to always be clean and well groomed. In public I expect them to wear dresses, together with flesh-coloured stockings, suspenders and shoes that have a heel. I appreciate that stilettos are not always practical, so anything over an inch and of any shape is acceptable. Boots may also be worn if the weather is cold. Dresses should button at the front or have been passed as acceptable by me, and should be knee-length or below. Submissives should strive to appear feminine at all times.

You will not wear a bra or panties when you are in my company unless by prior agreement.

Despite current fashions for shaving or waxing away pubic hair, I expect my submissives to be untrimmed and whole. In my opinion shaving or removing pubic hair infantilises women. This, for me, is not the same as consensual submission. I wish to share my life with adult women who are bright, communicative, mature and intelligent, and who have made an informed decision to submit sexually to their Master, to enjoy a BDSM lifestyle and defer to him in other areas of their life – which we will discuss if we decide to further our involvement. I do not need, nor do I expect you to be, a doormat.

However, I do expect you to be respectful and demure during our time together. I am the Master, you the submissive, and we are both here by choice rather than coercion, so if at any time you feel unhappy with my rules you are at liberty to leave.

During this first meeting you will refer to me as Sir. When our conversation can be overheard by other people you will refer to me as Mr Neal.

If you become part of my life then I shall expect you to have a full medical and be tested for STDs as I prefer unprotected sex.

There was more, but the nub of it was that Charles was another old-fashioned and very formal Dom, like Max, although I wasn't so sure about his rules. No make-up? Was the man mad? I looked like a chicken without a little eyeliner and mascara. How, once you got past twenty-five, could you strive to look feminine without at least a little cosmetic assistance? But Charles's profile and what he had written on a related web page and blog made interesting reading.

According to his profile he had not long turned fifty and had been in the lifestyle since he was in his mid-twenties. He was well educated, well read, gregarious, successful, and owned his own business. Charles was also clearly hot on contracts, rules and the way he expected his submissives to behave, which, given that this was what I was used to with Max, was one of the things that attracted me to him and his profile. He was most definitely old-school BDSM, and while Charles's rules appeared on the face of it to be, if anything, more rigid, I wasn't planning to live with him, so I was more or less certain that if we clicked I could cope with staying in role during the time we were together.

Before we met Charles had sent me a couple of photographs, but they didn't prepare me for the man himself. Charles was around five foot ten, with a mass of silver-grey hair that he wore brushed back off his face. He was built like a rugby player, with a great thick muscular neck, and was stocky with broad shoulders, big arms and thighs like tree trunks. None of it appeared to be fat. He watched me as I opened the café door and got to his feet as I approached the table, which was tucked away in an alcove.

He made me feel tiny.

'Sarah,' he said, catching my hand in his and shaking it firmly. 'I'm delighted that you could make it. Come, come –'

He pulled out a chair and indicated that I should sit down.

I'd found it very hard to go out without make-up on so had settled on a compromise: a bit of tinted moisturiser and some mascara. I wondered if Charles would notice.

As I settled myself into the seat, he waved the waitress over and then turned to face me. 'Tea?'

I nodded. 'Yes, please, Sir,' I said, taking a look around. The café was probably half full but where we were sitting – well away from the picture window that overlooked the main gardens – it was much quieter.

He smiled. 'Good, I'm glad you don't have a problem with addressing me correctly. I took the liberty of inviting a couple of the others to join us. I hope you don't mind.'

I did a double take, not sure that I had heard him correctly. '*The others?*' I said, in complete surprise.

He nodded. 'Yes, they're very excited about meeting you. Actually, it's because of them that you're here. Enid was the one who spotted your profile on the website. We've been looking for a while now.'

This wasn't what we had arranged. Two women, both without make-up, who had been sitting at the table across the room from where we were, now got to their feet and came over to join us.

'Sarah,' said Charles, 'this is Enid and Tania.'

They both smiled at me, both waiting for Charles to give them permission to sit down. Enid, the older of the two, was probably around my age, quite petite, with long auburn hair and fabulous skin and was dressed in a bohemian hippy fashion. She leaned over and kissed me on the cheek.

'Hello,' she said. 'I'm so glad you came. I'm dying to hear all about you, and your writing. I've always wanted to write.'

Tania followed suit. 'We wondered if you'd turn up,' she said conversationally, sliding her handbag onto one of the unoccupied chairs.

'We've had quite a lot of people stand Charles up,' said Enid.

Tania nodded. 'The problem is, I think a lot of woman like the fantasy element of a BSDM relationship but when it comes right down to it can't make the transition from there of turning it into a reality.'

'It is a big step,' said Enid, more kindly.

Tania rolled her eyes. 'Timewasters,' she said. She was dressed in a little floral number and a cardigan and looked like a nursery school teacher. She was younger than Enid by several years, probably in her early to mid thirties, taller and much curvier, with mousey blonde hair caught up in an ornate clip. Enid was wearing a long crushed-velvet dress and high-heeled sandals, along with a mass of African jewellery. She looked outdoorsy and fit as a flea.

Charles was watching me closely. 'Would you prefer it if we were alone?' he asked.

A bit late to ask me now, I thought. I was speechless. In his profile Charles had mentioned that he was interested in polygamy – the practice of having more than one wife, or in this case more than one submissive. It had been a fleeting reference, maybe a couple of lines, couched in terms of 'this would be my ideal set-up and I'm taking steps to try to make it a reality'. Charles had also said that he would like some of his polygamous subs to be bisexual. I just thought this was probably part of some complex fantasy – he certainly wouldn't be the first man I'd met who harboured a craving for a three-in-a-bed romp; I think a lot of men do, not just Doms – but I hadn't for one moment assumed it to be his everyday reality.

In my defence, lots of people on BDSM websites are fantasists and, while there is nothing wrong with that, it meant that, during the time I'd been meeting Doms, I'd tended to assume that at least some of what they told me was wishful thinking or exaggeration. So I had rather naïvely assumed that this was the case with Charles. It appeared that I was wrong.

'No, no, please,' I said, once I'd composed myself, looking up at the two women. 'Please, sit down.' I think I wanted them to feel comfortable, but also not to draw attention to us.

Charles smiled at me. 'That's my job,' he said, and indicated that they should sit. The two of them each pulled out a chair and Enid picked up the menu. 'Can we have cake?' she asked Charles.

'Oh God, yes,' said Tania, taking the second menu. 'Can we, Sir? I'm absolutely famished.'

Charles's expression softened and he laughed. 'Don't mind me,' he said, lifting his hands in mock surrender. 'I'm just their Dom,' he continued, addressing his remark to me. Then to Tania he said: 'Of course you can have cake. Would you like a sandwich too?'

She laughed. 'No, cake will be just fine.'

I nodded and listened while they chatted. It was obvious that Charles was very fond of the two of them, but I was totally on the back foot. I had been prepared for a lot of things, but I certainly hadn't been expecting a Dom and his harem.

Enid handed me the menu. 'What about you? What would you like, Sarah?'

I glanced at her. 'I'm not sure,' I said, unable to focus on the print.

'I'm so excited that you're a writer,' said Tania, glancing at Enid. 'What sorts of things do you write?'

'Romances mostly,' I said. 'And some erotica.'

'Oh really,' said Tania, eyebrows lifting. 'I'd love to read some of that.'

Enid, meanwhile, smiled back at me. 'Are you a bit shocked by us? You look a bit shocked.'

I nodded. 'I am. Just a bit.'

She laughed. 'I keep telling Sir that he should really say something before he meets someone. We always come with the Master when he's meeting a potential new member, don't we?'

'Sometimes we just sit and watch,' said Tania. 'You know, from a distance, because not everyone is happy meeting us straight off. But it's important for us, because we have to be able to get on with whoever he chooses.'

'Very important, otherwise it just doesn't work. And they have to know about us,' added Enid. 'This lifestyle means that we all have to be very honest about how we feel. There is no room for any of us to have other relationships without the others knowing.'

'I've told Sir that he should just put it in the advert,' said Tania, looking at Charles sternly. 'Make it perfectly clear right from the start. We already know there are women out there who would be interested.'

'There are websites,' said Enid, in answer to the question I suspect she saw on my face. 'Most of them are in the States, but there are some people in the UK too.'

'He should say something,' repeated Tania.

'He prefers to talk about it face to face,' said Enid. This was obviously a regular topic of debate.

I looked from woman to woman. Charles seemed happy to let them do the talking, which I suspected was another reason why he brought them along.

'We don't all live together,' Enid continued. 'We did discuss it initially, but everyone felt it would probably be too much. We all need some downtime and our own space. But we get together regularly in twos or threes. To play and to see each other and for social events.'

'And we always get together for birthdays and Christmas and for special occasions,' said Tania.

'Like anniversaries,' said Enid. 'We all have one. When we first joined.'

I could see the waitress coming our way with her pad and pencil.

'Officially joined,' corrected Tania.

'Sorry, Tania is right. Everyone has a trial period to see how they get on. And then, when you're ready to commit, Charles chooses a commitment date.'

'Are we ready to order yet?' asked the waitress. Apparently we were. Enid and Tania ordered afternoon tea for four, with sandwiches and scones. Tania hated scones, so there was a lot of good-natured banter while Tania scuttled off to look in the cabinet to choose what she wanted instead. It felt oddly like a strange family outing. Charles presided over the three of us, sitting at the head of the table like the lion among his pride.

'And then we all come together for the commitment ceremony,' Enid said.

'How many of you are there?' I asked conversationally, once the waitress had made her way back to the kitchen.

'Just three at the moment, but we used to have four,' said Enid.

'Four is a good number,' said Tania, as she came back and sat down at the table.

'Less friction with four,' added Enid. 'Even numbers seem to work out better.'

I noticed that Enid and Tania were both wearing plain silver rings on their wedding fingers. Tania was wearing a beaded choker and Enid had a discreet silver hoop around her neck. Enid saw me looking. 'We don't wear them until we've made a commitment,' she said, running the necklace around between her finger and thumb. 'We each get a ring and a collar.'

'The ring is engraved with the date,' said Tania, holding out her hand to show me.

'So who is missing?' I asked, unconsciously finding my eyes drawn to the empty chair.

'Jane,' said Enid. 'She was busy, and usually only one or two of us come along with Charles. It would be a bit overwhelming if all of us showed up together.'

I didn't like to say that it was pretty overwhelming as it was.

'And what about the one who left?'

'Lynsey,' said Charles. The women had been chatting so much that it came as quite a surprise to hear him interrupt. The women nodded.

'She didn't really fit in,' said Enid. 'Which was a real shame.'

Tania nodded her agreement. 'She was really nice.'

'I liked her,' said Enid wistfully. 'But she found it very hard to share Charles with the rest of us. It upset the balance.'

'It isn't easy to live like this. It's easy to feel threatened by the other subs,' said Tania. 'It's easy to feel like you're not getting your share.'

'You all bring different things to what we have,' said Charles, gently resting his hand on Tania's. 'And love isn't a finite thing. Loving one person doesn't mean you love another less. I would say that each relationship is very different and, if you would like to join us, Sarah, then you and I have to take the time to build that relationship. I try to spend time with each of my submissives on their own, so that we build something real beyond the physical. I share different things, different interests, with each of them. But I understand it can be hard for the women. There isn't any acceptable Western model for what we're doing. And it can be quite isolating.'

'In some ways, if it was just sex and BDSM it would be easier,' said Enid.

'Which is why we need each other to talk to,' said Tania. 'And another reason why we all need to get on.'

Enid nodded. 'And then friends and family want to meet your new boyfriend, and do things like go to weddings and parties or come and visit and that kind of thing.'

I glanced at Charles. He smiled at me. I wondered how he managed to deal with the physical needs of four women, let alone the emotional ones. He must be exhausted. No wonder he let them do the talking.

'And you have to be quite strong mentally,' Tania was saying. 'It's really easy to get jealous and think that one of the others is getting more of Charles than you are.'

'And sometimes they are, because they need support or are going through a difficult time,' added Enid.

They both nodded in unison. I knew without going any further that this wasn't for me, but I was curious.

'And it's not just about more sex; it's also about more of his time,' said Edith. 'Time to go out together, or just sit and be together.'

'Or go to the cinema or the theatre,' said Tania. 'I mean, we do do that, but it has to be fair. Sometimes we all go, but it can be tricky, especially if you want some time alone or you need time to talk about something but it's not your night or your time — if you see what I mean.'

I could see why Charles had brought the two of them along. They allayed any fears I had about him, and the more they talked the more I began to realise that for them it was a lifestyle that really worked. For me I knew that it wouldn't. In an emotional relationship I want to be the most important person in my partner's life, not one of many. I don't want to have my allotted time with him timetabled in, but for them it was obviously working.

'Each time someone new joins there is always a period of adjustment,' said Enid. 'And it takes a while for everything to settle down. Although the primary relationship is with Charles, we still all need to get along at some level. We've had a few false starts.'

'That's why it's important not to rush it,' said Tania. 'For a little while the new person destabilises what we've got —'

Enid nodded. 'Every time. And it's really hard to see someone you love falling in love with someone else.'

It was mind-boggling stuff. I glanced at Charles and realised that I wished he would talk more.

Tania, meanwhile, started to explain that she was a mature student and was living with Charles while she was doing her course; this was mainly because he lived within commuting distance of where she was studying. He was helping to fund her studies and in return she kept house for him and helped Enid. Enid worked as Charles's PA and lived in a house that Charles rented for her. The third sub,

Jane, also had a flat close to Charles – also paid for by him – and she was self-employed and worked from home. Today she was out meeting a client. The recent departure, Lynsey, had planned to work as a housekeeper and gardener for them all, but it hadn't worked out. They didn't expand too much on why, nor on how long Lynsey had lasted before deciding to bow out.

The tea and scones came and they chatted about shared projects – a garden they were building at Charles's house, a holiday cottage he had his eye on where they could all stay together for longer periods to see how it felt living as one big family – and the need to have their own space and time away from the intensity of polygamy. And the sex.

'Charles prefers to have two of us there at a time,' said Enid casually. 'Don't you, Sir?'

He nodded. 'I like to add a little spice where I can. And in the house I expect my submissives to be naked at all times or, alternatively, dressed as I instruct them.'

Tania smiled. 'You should come and see the house. There is the most fabulous dungeon. And a big dressing-up box.'

'And Jane and I are both bisexual,' said Enid conversationally, buttering her scone.

Driving home my mind busily raked over the afternoon's events. When I'd said, 'I don't really think this is for me,' Charles had suggested that I ought not to be so quick to dismiss the idea. He could, he said, offer me what I wanted: a caring relationship, BDSM and companionship. He would be happy to be my Master, and was a man who could embrace all the things that I was. I'd been so stunned by their arrangement that I hadn't really considered whether I found him attractive or not. The set-up was just so out of my comfort zone that I couldn't think of any set of circumstances which would ever make it a proposition I would seriously consider.

Even so, Charles suggested I didn't rush, that I should mull it over and give myself time to think, rather than hastily make a decision. Prospective candidates could join them on a three-month trial with no obligation. Enid and Tania had nodded and suggested that maybe I should come over and spend a weekend with them, meet Jane, maybe play a little, see how they lived and how it felt, and meet their pets.

I immediately thought about the man who liked to keep women in cages, but apparently they meant real pets: a goat, two dogs, some chickens and Enid's cats.

I promised that I would think about it, and I found that I *was* thinking about it, but perhaps not in the way they hoped for.

It wasn't that I was attracted to the idea – nor, if I'm honest, that I was shocked – so much as being surprised and interested by the notion of living a polygamous life. I don't think it would work for me; Enid said one of the main reasons she liked it was because she felt supported and never alone. She and Charles had been together for nearly ten years. They had begun with a Dom and sub relationship, Tania had joined them two years later and Jane had been with them for just over four years. It was obviously working for them.

Enid said part of the attraction was that she could always share what she felt. There were people around her who knew and understood Charles as well as she did, and who were in the BDSM lifestyle as well, and this made her life easier. None of the women had children, but Charles had a grown-up son and daughter. I didn't get into how that worked.

Charles saw himself as the hub of the wheel. I found it fascinating. We have such a closed view of what families and relationships are. Looking in from the outside, most people would have probably thought they were weird or that what they had was sordid, but it didn't feel like that at all. It felt like they were a family; strange and different, but a family nonetheless.

I also suspected from what they said that it wasn't easy being part of something so different from our cultural norms. Who did you talk to about it if it was going wrong, or share it with if it was going right? It was certainly food for thought, but most definitely not for me.

Just as I pulled up outside my house my mobile phone rang, but by the time I had negotiated parallel parking whoever it was had rung off.

Once I was back in the house I pulled my phone out of my handbag. One missed call. I scrolled down to see who it was and stared at the name on the screen. It was Max. Of all the people in the world who might ring me, he was the very last person I expected it to be. It unsettled me a little. It had been over a year since I had last seen him. Why was he ringing me now, after all this time? I flicked through to see if he had left a voicemail, but there was nothing.

Surely if he had wanted to talk to me then Max would have left a message, or asked me to call him back? Maybe he had called me by mistake. Easily done. Press the wrong button when you're scrolling through the phone book on your mobile ...

My phone rang again. This time the screen read: 'Caller Withheld'. I took a deep breath and let it ring for a second or two. Maybe Max thought I wouldn't answer if I knew it was him. Maybe ... I'd never find out unless I took the call.

'Hello?' I said tentatively.

'Hi, are you all right?' asked Gabbie.

'Oh, it's you,' I said, slumping down on the sofa.

'No need to sound so disappointed. I just wanted to know how your date went today. Are you okay? You sound really odd.'

Gabbie had been my safe call for my date with Charles, and I'd texted her when I was leaving to say I'd give her a ring as soon as I got home. But Gabbie wasn't as patient as that – trust her to get my arrival time down to within five minutes.

'I'm fine.'

'You don't sound it. How did it go?'

'Well, it was different,' I said. I had no intention of telling her about Enid and Tania showing up, nor about their unusual living arrangements.

'So that would be a no then, would it?'

'I'm afraid so,' I said. 'Another one off the list.'

'Oh, for God's sake! Why don't you just go out with Alex and be done with it? He sounds lovely. I don't see what the problem is.'

'Because –' I felt around for a reason and came up empty. 'I've got some other men I've been talking to,' I said.

'And they're going to be better, are they?' Gabbie said.

In reality, I knew Alex was going to be a hard act to follow, but I felt obligated to at least try. 'I've got no idea,' I said.

'Have you ever heard the old adage: better a bloke in the hand than two in the bush?'

I laughed.

'Anyway,' Gabbie went on, 'obviously I want all the details of what went wrong today, but first I want to know what you're planning to buy Joan as a wedding present.'

'She said she didn't want any presents.'

'Oh, come off it,' said Gabbie. 'Nobody doesn't want a present. She's just saying that to be polite. We have to get her something. We just need to work out what …'

'She told me if I bought her anything she would never speak to me again.'

'She's exaggerating. Who doesn't want a present?' said Gabbie.

'Joan, apparently.'

Gabbie sighed. 'There must be something we can get her.'

My invitation was still propped up on the mantelpiece. On the back of mine she had handwritten:

If you, Gabbie and Helen can't make it then I've told
Tom that I'll change the date so you can – I want you all
there to share our day. And don't feel you have to bring a
plus one, although you can if you want to – after all, I'm
bringing one.

'And what are you going to wear?' Gabbie was asking.

Joan and Tom were having a church wedding followed
by a barn dance; nothing I possessed was going to make
that transition without a change of shoes at the very least.

'And are you bringing anyone?' Gabbie wanted to know.

Helen would be bringing Geoff. Obviously.

'I've invited Alex, but I can put him off. We could go,
just us two,' I said. 'Girls together.'

'People will think we're gay,' said Gabbie. 'Remember
when we had that girls' weekend away and they gave us
two double rooms and when we said we weren't couples
and wanted single beds that woman in reception kept
saying, "We don't mind, we have nothing against gays"?'

I groaned. 'Okay, so who are you bringing?'

'I was thinking of maybe asking Dave.'

'You're seeing someone?' I said. It seemed like the rules
about vetting each other's men had now gone right out of
the window.

'No, he works at our place. He's been there since before
Christmas. He's an accountant. But that's not as bad as it
sounds. He's a hoot. And then if he goes, you can definitely
bring Alex.'

'It's only because you're nosey and want to meet him.'

'I want to see what's wrong with him.'

I sighed. 'There's nothing wrong with him.'

Which was when my landline started to ring. 'Hang on,' I said. 'I just need to see who this is.' I glanced at the number, wondering if Max might be trying again. But no. 'It's work,' I said. 'Can I call you back?'

'Don't worry. I'll ring later. I want to hear about today's date, but I've got a client about to come in. I'll ring you tonight. Talk soon. And think about Joan's present!'

It had been years since I had been in a church and I'd certainly never expected to find myself in the second pew from the front, along with Alex, Gabbie and Dave, and Helen and her new man, Geoff, all of us taking precedent over Joan's extended family, all of us dressed up to the nines and all of us eyeing up each other's plus ones. But Joan had made it perfectly clear that that was the way she wanted it. She had hung a sign on the end of the pew in her distinctive handwriting, reserving the pew just for us.

Alex was just fine – as I knew he would be – and was happily chatting away to Gabbie and Helen. Dave really was a hoot and quite obviously gay – if you didn't have a date to bring along to a do, he would be anyone's perfect plus one. And Helen's new man, Geoff? Well, he was pleasant, but quite quiet, and was obviously weighing us all up. I'm being charitable here. He watched us all with a look of quiet disapproval, and in all the years I've known her, Helen had never looked so gussied up, so bland, nor so very smoothed out. There is no way in a million years she would have chosen those shoes on her own. She kept glancing at him to make sure he was all right, and both of them looked uncomfortable. Having known and loved her for so long, it was painful to watch.

'Maybe he'll thaw out once he gets to know us,' said Gabbie, out of the corner of her mouth.

'Let's hope so,' I whispered. It's awkward when you don't hit it off with your friend's partner and they very obviously don't approve of you, but moving on …

Tom, Joan's groom, was a great big man with a beard who swooped on us the moment we arrived. I could see in an instant exactly why Joan was so certain he was the one. He hugged all of us, great big bear hugs, and giggled about trying to find a suit to fit. He chatted about Joan and the palaver over the music and the dress and made us feel in moments as if we had known him for years, and that Joan getting married was not the seismic shift I think we had all feared. His best man was the caller in the ceilidh band and was desperate to get out of his suit and back into his dancing shoes. He had a pigtail that reached almost to his waist and an extremely impressive moustache.

Joan's children were in the row in front of us, all grown up now and with their respective partners. It had been years since I'd seen them, so it was lovely to catch up.

The church was full and bubbling with conversation and laughter. We all knew that Joan was popular in the village and in her church, but I don't think any of us had realised just how popular. And then the music started. The opening bars stilled the congregation, and into the vast silence came the strains of something lush and classical. We all turned to watch Joan come down the aisle, squired by her eldest son. They walked slowly, waving and smiling and acknowledging the guests.

Joan was glowing. I know it's a cliché, but she looked amazing, like an intense, polished, extra-beautiful version of herself. Joan is quite tiny and when I'm away from her I always forget that she is so petite. For her wedding she wore a cream coat suit and a hat with a veil and carried a bouquet of cream roses. Actually, it doesn't do her justice to say that she looked beautiful; it was much, much more than that. She had a big smile on her face and before I knew what was happening, tears of absolute joy were rolling down my face.

I glanced up the aisle towards Tom, who was waiting for Joan to arrive. He, too, had the biggest, happiest smile you could ever see and, as they got closer, they only had eyes for each other. I realised as their gaze met that at that moment none of us really mattered, even though everyone there wanted nothing more than to share their day with them. The look they exchanged was so tender, so full of love and delight, you'd have to have been made of stone not to be touched by it. If ever proof was needed that love wasn't just the preserve of the young and perky, this was it. As she got to the steps of the nave, Tom took her hand and his smile grew wider still. It touched my heart to see them so obviously happy, and I couldn't help wondering if anything that wonderful would ever happen to me.

Sitting next to me, Alex gently squeezed my hand, while Gabbie did the same on the other side. Just beyond her, Dave was sobbing like a baby. Helen was crying too.

Only Geoff stared fixedly ahead. I'm not sure whether he was embarrassed by the rest of us or just trying to hold it together. Or perhaps he wasn't touched by it at all.

The vicar welcomed us all and then began the service.

'We are gathered here today to witness the wedding of Joan and Tom,' he said, smiling out into the congregation. I was completely lost in the moment. I've been to lots of church weddings in my life, but this one, between one of my oldest friends and her new man, was so touching and so heartfelt that the words I'd heard dozens of times before took on a new and special significance.

I think Gabbie, Dave, Helen and I cried more or less the whole way through. My carefully applied make-up was ruined after the first five minutes, while Alex, bless him, just kept handing round the tissues.

After the ceremony we all headed off to the reception and barn dance, Gabbie, Dave and I taking time out to change into jeans and sensible shoes in the loo. Dave changed into a cowboy shirt and string tie; Alex took his tie off. Gabbie found us a table. We danced all evening, long into the night, and ate, drank and generally had a fine old time.

The only real downside was that at around eight o'clock Helen announced that she and Geoff had to leave as they were picking up his grandson from somewhere or other, which seemed a terrible shame. Gabbie couldn't understand why they were leaving so early – surely a best friend's wedding took precedence over picking up a teenager from youth club, but we all suspected that it was because Geoff wanted to make an early getaway and needed an excuse. It was a shame they had to go, but it didn't dampen our spirits for too long.

'Thank you for inviting me,' said Alex, as we careered around the dance floor arm in arm. As we got to the end of the line of eight people who were taking part in our bit of the folk dance, he spun me around.

I grinned. 'Thank you for coming. Not exactly a night of wild BDSM, though, is it?'

'I'm not sure I'll have the energy after this,' he said breathlessly, as we sidestepped back down through the dancers.

I giggled. 'No stamina.'

He pulled me in close and kissed me hard. 'You'll pay for that later.' Under the instructions from the caller, we lifted up our hands to form an arch and everyone skipped under it.

'I thought you said you didn't have the energy?' I said.

'I'm keeping a tally,' he said. 'It might not be tonight, but you will most certainly pay for being cheeky.'

'Promise?' I teased.

'That's two now,' Alex said, as the music finally stopped and we staggered back to our table. 'Do you want another drink?' I nodded.

While he went off to the bar, I sat down and caught my breath.

'He's lovely,' said Gabbie, sliding in alongside me. 'I don't know what you were worried about or why you haven't snapped him up.'

I looked up towards the bar and smiled; she was right.

'I know. But I've got six months,' I said.

Gabbie raised her eyebrows. 'What, so that you can make up your mind? And see other people?'

I nodded.

She sniffed. 'Are you mad? How would you feel if Alex was seeing someone?'

I stared at her. 'He isn't.'

'So you say, but how would you feel?'

'I'd hate it.'

She nodded. 'Maybe Alex does too.'

'It was his idea, not mine,' I said.

'I'm just saying I wouldn't leave it too long, that's all. Not if you're sure.'

'That's my problem. I'm not.'

'Oh for fuck's sake,' said Gabbie, sounding frustrated. 'You only have to see you two together to know that you're perfect for each other. There's no helping some people.'

When the party was finally over and we'd cut the cake, drunk all the champagne and waved goodbye to the bride and groom, Alex and I took a cab back to the tiny bed and breakfast I'd booked us into. It was in a farm cottage and we had a double room in a tiny annexe that had once been stables. Both drunk on the atmosphere and the champagne, we tumbled into bed and spent the night curled up in each other's arms.

BDSM? Not in any sense of the narrowest definition. But that sense of being his, and of Alex being in control, was there all the time; the feeling of being with a strong alpha male, easy in his own skin without being arrogant, a man who knew how to take care of a woman, was and still is for me the mark of a true Dom.

We woke up early, the morning sun streaming in through the window in the roof of our room.

As I yawned and stretched, Alex reached across to the bedside table and took out a small gift-wrapped box from the drawer. 'I've bought you a little something,' he said, handing it to me.

I shook it speculatively. Nothing moved, nothing rattled. Whatever was inside it was either well wrapped or filled the whole box.

'Aren't you going to open it?' Alex asked. 'We've got time to try them out before breakfast.'

Very carefully I peeled away the outer wrapping. Inside was a pair of stainless-steel handcuffs, proper police handcuffs, the chain wrapped with tissue so that it hadn't moved when I'd shaken it.

'What do you think?' said Alex, eyes bright.

I held out my hands, wrists together. 'I'll come quietly officer,' I said.

He grinned. 'I've got a ball gag in my bag, so you can come as noisily as you like,' he said.

So why didn't I just carry on seeing Alex after that? It's a question that, looking back now, still puzzles me. It would have made perfect sense. Anyway, he was the most perfect plus one to take to the wedding, and the best fun the morning after.

The things that Gabbie had said did strike a chord, but I still couldn't bring myself to call it a day on my Dom search. Although, madly, it wasn't like I wasn't seeing him at all. I just wasn't seeing him exclusively.

We still had his posh event booked in the diary, but I felt perfectly fine about getting back to my search for the right Dom.

# Chapter Eleven

Of all the men I've met over the years on internet dating sites, the Doms on the BDSM sites I've visited have been among some of the nicest and most interesting, but there is always an exception to the rule, and part of the problem with Danny was that I broke my own rules right from the very start.

'We're going to get on so well,' Danny said jokily, when we spoke on the telephone. It was late and we'd been on the phone for most of the evening, talking about our lives, our interests beyond BDSM and generally putting the world to rights; the time had just flown by.

'Sometimes you can just tell, don't you think?' he said. Danny had sent me his profile a few weeks earlier and we had emailed back and forth a few times before progressing to instant messenger and then to phone calls.

Danny told me that he was on garden leave from a job in the City. He was well educated, liked skiing and rugby and had, he said, done well for himself after a shaky start. When I asked him what he meant by that, he said his mother had been ill for most of his childhood and initially he had really struggled at school.

'My parents were separated, I was going to this little school in the village where my mother lived ... Anyway, then I went off to boarding school,' he said brightly. 'I suppose I was seven or eight. My grandfather thought it would be a good idea and he was right. Suddenly, once I was away from it all, my life really came together.'

'That's brilliant. And how about your mum?'

'She's up and down, but it's much easier now that I'm an adult. I can get some distance, you know? She's never really going to be well, but she copes,' he said, sounding keen to move on from the subject. We talked about parents and life and how much he loved his grandparents and what a stabilising factor they had been in his life. We talked about art and music and how he liked to paint and wanted to write. We talked about BDSM and what we were both looking for.

'Did you get the photos I just sent you?' he asked.

I most certainly had. They had arrived as we had been speaking and I'd just clicked on the email attachments and opened up the images.

'So?' he said. 'What do you think?'

What did I think? 'They're great photos,' I said cautiously.

Danny was younger than me by about eight years, and if the photos were anything to go by he had boyish good looks, along with a mop of floppy brown hair and huge brown eyes. In one of the photos he was at the zoo and had a little girl sitting up on his shoulders. He was holding onto her legs and looking up at her while she smiled shyly for the camera. He told me she was the daughter of a friend.

'I used to babysit for her a lot when she was tiny,' he said. 'Her name is Sophie and she is an absolute poppet.

She's grown so much since that photo. You wouldn't believe –'

The second picture was of Danny with two Labrador puppies in a garden. He was sitting on the grass and wearing a denim shirt and jeans. One of the puppies was standing up on its back legs, paws on his arm, licking his face. Danny was pulling away from the long pink tongue, but was nonetheless laughing at the camera. The third and final photo was a moody, atmospheric studio shot.

'A friend of mine suggested that I ought to try modelling,' he said casually. 'So I had these done for my portfolio. It cost me a fortune, but it was fun to do. I thought I might as well get some use out of them. So, what do you think? Don't laugh.'

I most certainly wasn't planning on laughing. 'They're lovely, and the professional one is fabulous,' I said.

It was shot in black and white and beautifully lit. Danny was sitting on a stool against an all-white backdrop and was naked to the waist. He was wearing skinny black jeans and was turned in three-quarter profile towards the camera; his hair was wet and mussed up. He was wiping himself dry with a bright-white towel. He had a broad, almost perfectly symmetrical hairless chest and even broader swimmer's shoulders, along with big upper-arm muscles and a six-pack. His muscles were beautifully defined, as were his cheekbones, which were emphasised by just a hint of designer stubble. To get into that sort of shape and to stay that way must take a lot of effort. It was a beguiling, striking and very sexy photo.

'Did you get any work?' I asked.

'No. In the end I didn't think it was quite my thing.'

'They're really good. I'm surprised you didn't get snapped up.'

He laughed. 'Maybe I'll give it another go some time. As I said, not quite my thing.'

Looking at the images, my first thought was that Danny wasn't quite *my* thing. In all truth I thought he was probably out of my league. And before anyone squeals in protest, I'm not being self-deprecating or putting myself down; Danny was just not the sort of man who would usually give me a second look. And more telling was the fact that I wouldn't usually look at him, either. He was pretty rather than handsome, boyish rather than manly, and probably spent longer in the bathroom getting ready than I did. Put simply, he was not my type. But Danny was insistent that we would get on really well, and on the phone he was charming, funny, sexy and good company. Maybe he was right, but –

'I think you look great, but I'm not really sure,' I began.

'Oh come on, Sarah. At least give me a chance,' he said. 'What's the problem?'

Here was a man who looked as if he had just stepped out of the pages of a fashion magazine, asking *me* to give *him* a chance. I wondered briefly whether the BDSM thing might level the playing field, but I knew that it wouldn't. It wasn't enough in my book. I needed to be comfortable and at ease with my Dom. There were lots of younger, far more beautiful women out there who I suspected would be only too happy to be tied up and tormented by someone as attractive as Danny.

And he looked like the kind of man who would be more attracted to them than to someone who was over forty with grown-up children. When I pointed this out to Danny, he laughed it off. Even so, I felt like there was something that wasn't quite right, but I decided to ignore my instincts. After all, what did they know? Weren't these the same instincts that told me I should be having my happy-ever-after with Alex?

'Most of my partners have been older than me,' Danny said, when I pressed him. 'My first serious girlfriend was eight years older than me, my ex-wife was ten years older. I don't know what it is; I suppose I just prefer more mature women, that's all. I like the fact that they're usually more confident, more at ease with themselves and their sexuality. Particularly when it comes to BDSM. In my experience, younger women who other people may think of as pretty can often be shallow, and they're just playing at it. You know, they haven't really had to try to be anything or anybody – their looks have just opened doors for them. No, I prefer my women with some depth and experience. I much prefer their company. I want a book, not a magazine.'

Danny was saying all the right things, but I still wasn't totally convinced.

'You mean older women are grateful,' I joked.

'Well, there is that,' he said.

I laughed. He laughed.

'There are things I like to do that I don't think a younger woman could appreciate or maybe even cope with,' he said.

'Like what?' I asked warily.

'Nothing that weird. I like to objectify my sub while we're playing – I like the idea of my partner being there purely for my pleasure, just a sex toy. But obviously we agree the limits beforehand,' he said hastily. 'And I like name-calling, referring to my subbie by what might be considered an abusive name: slut or whore – or worse –'

None of these things were out of the ball park as far as I was concerned.

'And of course I'd like to push you to your limits, but not until we get to know each other better.'

'So we can take it slowly?' I asked.

He laughed. 'If you insist. But I think once we meet up you'll be fine and won't want to take it slowly at all.'

'I reserve the right to go slowly,' I said.

'Of course,' he said.

By the time we got to the end of the phone call, we'd agreed that we'd like to meet up, despite my reservations. After all, what was there to lose?

Which was where the trouble started. Since his divorce, Danny said, he'd been sharing a house with friends, so we couldn't meet at his place. I pointed out that this was jumping the gun a bit. Even if he had a house, I wouldn't be meeting him there. Not for a first meeting. We should meet somewhere public, I said.

Danny was amused. 'Why?' he asked, sounding genuinely surprised that I'd suggested it.

'Have you met women from the website before?'

'A few.'

'And you met them at their homes?'

'Yes, and when I didn't we went for a drink first and then went back to her flat.'

I didn't want to judge how other women conducted their meetings, but I reserved the right to arrange mine so that I felt comfortable. 'I'd prefer it if we met on neutral territory to begin with.'

He laughed. 'Okay, that's not a problem, but tell me why.'

'So we both feel safe, and so that if we don't get on or we're not attracted to each other, we can just smile, have a cup of coffee and go our separate ways. How many people have you met from the website so far?'

I can't remember if Danny answered me or not. I think not, but I do remember him saying, 'Oh come on, like that's going to happen. We get on so well on the phone.'

'So suggest somewhere,' I said.

'I don't drive,' he said. 'Tell you what, why don't I come to you? I could come down on the train.'

Every other time someone had suggested meeting me in my home town I had politely but firmly declined. Up until Danny, I had always met men in anonymous, safe public places – usually cafés and restaurants away from home. I also knew that Danny didn't just mean my home town; what he really meant was that he wanted to come to my home. But this time I ignored my usual rules and said: 'Yes, okay, why not?' After all, we'd been talking for a while, he looked harmless and he sounded great – and I was flattered. I was stupid ...

Over the course of the conversation our plans firmed up. Danny would come down by train, we'd have lunch somewhere quiet in town where we could chat. I'd pick him up at eleven and take him back to the station at around half past two or three o'clock.

'We'll need to check the timetable for return trains,' he said. 'Unless of course we hit it off, and then who knows what time I'll leave?' Danny purred.

I didn't comment. I'd been on so many dates where a Dom and I had got on really well over the phone but there had been no chemistry when we met up that I didn't like to second-guess the outcome.

Before he hung up Danny said: 'I want you to call me Sir when we meet.'

'Fine,' I said. It was common currency between Dom and sub, and I knew that I wouldn't find it hard to do. But Danny hadn't finished with his instructions.

'And when you come to the station I want you to wear stockings and suspenders, high heels and nothing else. I want you to be naked under your coat. I'll be thinking about you all the way there ... Oh, and don't wear anything that's too long. I'm thinking it would be sexy to get a flash of stocking top as you walk across the platform to meet me.'

I laughed; this was well beyond my limits on a first date. 'No way, José. And it's my local railway station we're talking about here, Danny. People know me.'

'Who is the Dom here?' asked Danny, sounding amused. 'You'll live to regret disobeying me, Sarah. I plan to punish you. You know that, don't you?'

'Let's see how we get on first, shall we?' I said flippantly. I was getting used to Doms posturing and announcing their intentions. It was part of the game and added a little frisson of expectation and excitement. And then Danny said something odd. He said: 'I'm sure you and I will get on very well, because I'm an impressive man. I find that a lot of people are impressed by me. I think people find me intimidating.'

We made some joke about it, but it stuck with me.

A few days later I was sitting in my car outside the railway station waiting for Danny's train to arrive. The plan we'd settled on was that I'd pick him up from the train station and then we'd go for lunch at a nice little country pub about half an hour's drive away. It was fairly close to home, but not too close. I also knew very well that Danny was planning to try to persuade me that it might be more fun to go straight back to mine to play. I wasn't altogether against the idea, but I planned to wait and see how I got on with him; I was in no hurry to rush into anything and certainly not to take him home to my cottage.

The train was a little late, so while I was waiting I texted Alex.

'So how's it going?' he texted straight back.

'Fine. I'm out to lunch today with another potential Dom.'

'Be much easier if you just gave in and realised that I'm Mr Right.'

'Lol – oh really, Mr Right?'

'That's Master Right, Sir, to you. Where are you going?'

'Why?'

'I might just pitch up and make a scene. Tell him you're already taken.'

'No way am I telling you in that case.'

'I'm at home,' he wrote. 'I could be your safe call, if you like.'

'Thanks, but I've got Gabbie on the case.'

'Okay, well, have a good time. Let me know how it goes and whether I should put my profile back up on the site.'

'You've taken it down?' I asked, genuinely surprised.

'Obviously.'

I heard the warning claxon that announced the barriers were coming down and the train was on its way.

'You didn't have to do that,' I typed.

'No, you're right, I didn't, but I did. So where are you going for lunch?'

I could see the train. 'I'm not telling you and I've got to go.'

'Enjoy. Talk to you later, assuming you're not too tied up.'

I typed 'Lol' and then pressed send.

The train slowed and pulled to a halt. A moment or two later the passengers began to disembark. I got out, locked the car and climbed the steps that would take me across the bridge over the lines to the far-side platform. Going against the flow of people heading for the exit slowed my progress. I quickly spotted Danny below me waiting on the platform. He was looking around among the rapidly dissipating crowd. He was dressed in a cream trench coat and was carrying a briefcase and wearing a trilby, which, along with what looked like cavalry twills and brogues, made him look like something out of a 1940s black-and-white movie. He was stretching up, craning his neck, looking left and right. I smiled to myself. If anything, he was better looking than in his photographs, and there was a real lithe energy in the way he moved.

I hurried down the steps and at the same time he turned towards me. When he spotted me and our eyes met, something about Danny's expression stopped me dead in my tracks and made my breath catch in my throat. I can't tell you exactly what it was; it was hard to define, but whatever it was, it set alarm bells ringing. I slowed my pace, gathering my thoughts. He was smiling and lifted a hand in greeting, but his gesture and expression looked false and mad. That was it – he looked mad, totally deranged. His eyes were bright and his smile looked more like a crazy, fixed grimace.

Short of abandoning Danny on the platform, I couldn't see what choice I had but to go up and speak to him. Before I opened my mouth he leaned in closer and grabbed the top of my arm so tightly that I winced.

'Where the hell have you been?' he said in a tight, angry voice, the strange rictal grin remaining in place. 'You understood my instructions, didn't you? I told you to be here waiting for me, didn't I? Here on the platform so that I could see what I was getting. I don't need you to make an entrance, is that clear? And I don't like to be kept waiting.' His fingers tightened and I flinched.

'I was just waiting in the car,' I said, extricating myself from his grasp. I tried to smile and look pleased to see him, in an effort to ease the tension. 'That hurt,' I said, rubbing my arm and stepping away from him, but he stepped straight back into my personal space.

'It was meant to. Isn't that what we're both looking for? Pain?' he snarled.

I tried out a smile.

'So you think it's funny, do you?' he continued.

'No, of course not,' I said. 'I'm just pleased you got here safe and sound,' I lied, hoping to appease him, while trying to work out how to get away from him.

In many ways this was the wake-up call I'd been dreading since I started looking for a Dom. The fact was that I'd become complacent about meeting a stream of strange men. And standing there on the platform with Danny, all the times I had convinced myself that my rules would keep me safe came back to haunt me. Danny seemed unstable. I most certainly wasn't going to get into a car with him, let alone take him back to my place – or anywhere else if I could possibly help it. Taking him home had been my idle fantasy as I'd flicked through his profile and photos. But now I didn't trust him enough to drive him anywhere. I needed a rapid rethink.

'The fucking train was late,' he snapped, still staring round. 'Where is this place we're going for lunch? I am starving. I need to eat.'

'Okay,' I said, still trying to come up with a plan. 'It's not far.'

Despite us being in a public place, Danny made me feel vulnerable. In all the time I'd been online dating I had never felt like this. And worse still, I knew that my strategy for staying safe was, in reality, close to useless. My rules only worked because all of the men I'd met up with until now were prepared to play by them.

'Why do you keep smiling?' Danny asked, between gritted teeth. 'I don't see anything remotely funny about this.'

'No, of course it's not funny,' I said, in my most reasonable voice, settling my face into a more neutral expression. 'Not at all. I think it's terrible the train was late and I appreciate that you're hungry.' My mind was working overtime. 'It's nice to meet you after all this time talking.'

'Is it?' he said. 'I thought you didn't want to meet me? I thought you thought I was too young – not your kind of thing. So, what do you think now?' He struck a pose.

I hesitated. 'Very impressive,' I said, remembering what he had told me on the phone. 'I think you're impressive.'

He nodded, the strange unnatural smile returning. 'I told you I'm impressive, and a lot of women can't handle it, you know. They've told me. They find me intimidating to be with.'

I nodded, not sure that there was an answer to this and desperate not to provoke him.

'I'm hungry,' he repeated.

I nodded again, trying hard to come up with something that would keep him out of my car.

The station, on the western edge of the town, is a brisk ten-minute walk from the town centre. On the station side of the town, in the main shopping parade, is an old pub where the food is reasonable and more importantly I know the people who own it – not well, as I'd only been living in the town for a couple of years, but well enough to feel confident that if anything happened there would be people there who would help me. I didn't know what it was I feared Danny might do, but my guess was that he could be unpredictable, probably aggressive and very possibly violent.

I closed my eyes, imagining just how potentially disastrous the next couple of hours could be. My private life, which I valued so very much, could be blown open in an instant if Danny turned nasty and made a scene. I imagined trying to explain how I had met him and why. It didn't bear thinking about.

'I just need to go and park my car,' I said. 'The restaurant's not far from here. In town. There's a shuttle bus that goes up into town every ten minutes or so, or we could walk.' I made the effort to sound warm and cheerful.

Danny peered at me. 'You're expecting me to get on a *bus?*' he said incredulously.

I nodded. 'The parking is really bad in town.' *Any excuse would do.* There was no way I wanted to be alone in a car with him.

'We'll get a taxi. I'm not getting on a fucking bus and I'm certainly not bloody walking.'

'Okay, well, I'll go and park the car and see if I can track down a taxi,' I said.

The main station forecourt is quite small. Usually when the trains pulled out of the station the taxis headed back into town with their fares, or if they hadn't picked anyone up left to look for richer pickings. Not that I told Danny that. I just wanted to get away from him.

'And what am I supposed to do while you're gone. Why don't I come with you?' he said.

Thinking quickly, I said: 'Why don't you see if they do a complaints form. For the train being late. I'll only be a few minutes. They probably have a form in the ticket office.'

Danny nodded and walked back with me over the bridge, holding tightly onto my arm every step of the way. I took a deep breath and tried very hard to stay calm. His grip and his closeness was unnerving. 'There's no need to hold onto me like that,' I said, in a neutral but fairly firm voice.

'I like the way it feels, and I want you to call me Sir. We agreed that you would.'

'You're right, we did, Sir. Did you have a good journey?' I asked, still trying to ease the tension and keep him calm and reasonable.

'No. There was some moron with his iPod on the whole way. I told him – I said, if he didn't want me to smash the fucking thing he'd better turn it down.'

I nodded. Danny's anger, his frustration, whatever this volatility was, bubbled darkly just beneath the surface. Even now I can't work out how he managed to keep it hidden while we were talking on the phone. We talked for hours. I've replayed those conversations over and over in my head, and up until the strange remark about him being impressive, there had been nothing to make me think that he was anything other than ordinary and pleasant and potentially good company. There was certainly never any inkling that he had any kind of mental-health issues.

We were almost at the ticket office, which was in the building on the way out to the car park. 'There we are. The ticket office is just there,' I said brightly, pointing, while easing myself out of his grasp. 'See you outside.'

Danny let go of me and appeared to head off in the direction I'd pointed to, while I practically ran back to the car, unlocked it and jumped in. I was just reversing back from where I was parked when I saw Danny in my mirrors, standing behind the car. He must have more or less followed me straight out. Instinctively – certainly without thinking about the consequences – I slammed on the brakes.

Within in what seemed like an instant he was round by the passenger-side door and I wasn't quick enough or bright enough to drive away. 'I'll do it when I get home,' he said, pulling open the car door and climbing in.

'Right, okay,' I said, trying to keep the panic out of my voice. 'Well, in that case, we just need to park.'

'Why don't we just drive into town?'

'I already explained,' I began. I didn't add that I had been hoping to give him the slip.

'Stop,' Danny snapped, holding up a hand to silence me. 'Just stop here.' I realised that he meant the car.

'I can't stop here,' I said evenly. 'This is a drop-off and pick-up zone.'

'I know, but we haven't said hello properly yet, have we?' Danny said, and with that he launched himself at me. He kissed me hard on the mouth, sliding his hand up between my knees, which I instinctively nipped together. The car stalled.

He pulled away, wiping his mouth and laughing. 'You're a bit tense, aren't you? Jesus, I told you I intimidate people, or is it just that you're frigid?' His tone was jokey, but there was something altogether more unpleasant beneath it.

I smiled. 'I'm just a bit flustered, that's all,' I said.

'I can have that effect on people,' Danny replied. 'You need to learn how to relax. I can help you with that. I did a course.'

Without thinking I undid my coat so that I could manoeuvre the car more easily and was just pulling away when Danny leant over and grabbed the back of my neck. As I tried to push him away he leant across me and bit my breast as hard as he could – I screamed in pain as his teeth sank into me.

'Get off me! Get out of the car,' I said, thrusting him away. 'Get out, now! *Now!*'

'What?' Danny said, jerking away from me. 'What's the matter with you? I told you I was going to punish you for refusing to show up naked, didn't I? That was it. Isn't that what you want?'

'No,' I said. 'No, it isn't.' I was trembling. 'It was bloody dangerous to grab me while I was driving, never mind how hard you bit me. I want you to get out of my car. Now.'

He shrugged, the crazed look in his eyes apparently receding – not that I was at all fooled. I'd seen what was in there.

'Oh for fuck's sake, come on, Sarah,' said Danny. 'Lighten up. I'm sorry, all right? Was that too much too soon? I'm sorry, really, I am. Come on, relax. I thought that was what you wanted. Look, let's just go and eat, shall we? I apologise, all right? I didn't mean to frighten you or hurt you or whatever the fuck it was I did, okay? What more can I say? I thought you wanted me to stay in character. I'm good at it, you've got to admit, all that heavy Dom stuff. What do you think?'

I stared at him. Nothing he said could persuade me that what I'd just seen was an act.

'I'm famished,' he said. 'I'm always cranky when I'm hungry. Please, I'm really sorry. Let's start over, shall we? Friends?' He tipped his head to one side and batted his eyelashes, as if that might convince me. It was a horrible caricature of cute.

I needed Danny out of the car. If I couldn't get him out I would be trapped with him inside our own private little bubble, and even though there were people around I didn't feel safe – anything could happen. The station forecourt was emptying. I put the car in reverse and very slowly manoeuvred us out of the drop-off zone and into the main car park. I moved very deliberately, my hands tight on the wheel, terrified that he might try to grab me or the wheel while I was driving.

In the passenger seat, Danny was giggling. 'I really had you going there, didn't I? I thought I'd come over all Lord and Master and see how you liked it. You liked it, didn't you? You have to admit it, you really like that kind of thing. I can't get over the fucking train being late. Today of all days.' As he spoke he opened the glove compartment and started rifling through the contents.

'What are you doing?' I said.

'Looking for something to eat. Have you got anything to eat in here? Like chocolate or something?'

'No, not in there, but once we get parked we can go and get something.'

'Good,' he said, 'because I'm hungry.' And then Danny looked at me with a huge grin on his face. 'And you won't like me when I'm hungry,' he said.

My heart lurched. I didn't like him at all, hungry or not.

Even while I was trying to work out what to do next, I was berating myself for being so naïve. I had been so very smug about my stupid safe calls. When it came right down to it, I could be dead before anyone called out the cavalry. I drove round to the car park. At this time of the day there were several empty spaces. I pulled into the one that was nearest to the gate, manoeuvring into a bay alongside a middle-aged couple who were busy loading cases into their car. I wanted to stay as close to other people as I could.

'I just need to get a ticket from the machine,' I said, opening the car door and grabbing my handbag from the foot well.

'Don't be long,' said Danny. 'I'll be waiting for you.'

That was what was worrying me. I clambered out of the car and hurried across the car park. My phone was tucked in the top of my bag. I bent down, pretending to rootle around for my purse, and scrolled down to Alex's number and pressed dial. *'Hurry up, hurry up,'* I murmured under my breath, praying that he would pick up quickly. He did.

'So, stand you up, did he?' asked Alex. I don't think I've ever been so happy to hear anyone's voice. It was all I could do not to burst into tears.

'No, listen,' I said, still hunched over, still pretending to search for my purse. 'He's completely nuts.' Despite my best efforts I couldn't keep the emotion out of my voice. 'Please come, Alex, I'm frightened. I'm going to take him to The Crown and Mitre on the High Road.'

'I'm on my way,' he said, and hung up. The sense of relief was astonishing, although I still had to keep Danny calm and reasonable until Alex arrived.

I stood up and looked back towards the car. I was worried that Danny might have been watching me, but instead he was hunched over as if he was looking at something in the foot well.

I slipped the money into the machine and took out the ticket. I paid for four hours. It was four hours until Danny had agreed to leave. It was going to take Alex around forty minutes to get to the pub; all I had to do was hold it together for another forty minutes. The pain from the bite mark on my breast was stunning. I could feel it throbbing.

There were lots of ways I could have played this, but on the way back to the car I decided the best way to get rid of Danny and keep a lid on things was to go through the motions of it just being a normal meeting. I'd do my best to chat to him, keep him calm, keep him sweet and, whether Alex showed up or not, just get Danny back on the train and out of my life as soon as possible. I also vowed never to be so stupid or naïve again. That was the plan ...

When I got back to the car Danny rolled down his window. 'Get in,' he said. 'I thought we could go for a drive. I've never been to this part of the world before. I thought you could show me around.'

I made the effort to smile. 'But I've just bought a parking ticket, and besides, I thought you said you were hungry?'

'We could find somewhere on the way. A country pub or something. I fancy a little trip out. We can talk while you're driving. Get to know each other better.'

I said nothing and did nothing to indicate that I would be getting back in the car with him. After a moment or two he wound up the window, stretched and climbed out. 'What are you playing at? For a sub you're not very obedient, are you?' he said. 'You really do need someone to train you. To really take you in hand. Or do you like acting the brat?'

'No, of course not,' I said. 'It's just that it's easier to eat here in town. Somewhere I know.'

Danny pulled a face. 'Unadventurous, aren't you? I'll have to cure you of that. Bring you into line. That's what Doms do, don't they? I can see why you need one. Now, where is the fucking taxi rank?'

He looked round, scanning the area in front of the station.

I went to lock up the car. I wasn't aware that Danny was following me round to my side of the car, but as I turned from sorting out the keys he was almost on top of me and went to grab my arm.

'Get off me!' I said, all pretence of trying to be civil evaporating as I pushed him away.

He stepped back and then, as he regained his balance, he slapped me round the face. Hard. So hard that it made my head ring. I hadn't seen it coming. I was so stunned, so outraged, that I couldn't speak. This wasn't BDSM, or Ds. This was abuse. This was assault. And this was enough.

I stepped away from him, my cheek smarting, my eyes filling up with tears – not from being upset, although I was, but from the pain and the shock and the sheer unexpectedness of what Danny had just done. I struggled to breathe. This was crazy. If anyone had noticed what had just happened, they didn't come rushing over to rescue me. I was also furious. No one had ever done anything like that to me before and I had no intention of letting him think it was okay. I thought from his body language that there was a damned good chance he planned to hit me again, but I wasn't planning to back down. Stupid? Probably. But nonetheless, and really without thinking, instead of crumpling up, I stood up straight and looked Danny in the eyes.

'What the hell do you think you're doing?' I snapped.

He broke eye contact the instant it was made. 'Too much?' he asked.

'Way too much,' I said, feeling my anger grow. 'That's it, Danny, you need to go now.'

He stared at me. 'What do you mean? I've only just got here.'

'This meeting is over. Finished. You understand?'

Danny laughed and held up his hands as if totally bemused. 'Oh come on, Sarah. What's your problem? I thought you'd like it. It was just part of the game. I can tone it down, if you like, but you need someone like me in your life to make you understand what obedience means. I could teach you. I'm good at this. We could have fun.'

I wanted to tell Danny what I thought of his idea of fun, that for me this wasn't any kind of BDSM, that this was something madder and more dangerous and abusive and not at all what I wanted to be involved in, but I didn't intend to provoke him. I didn't even want to talk to him, let alone engage in a conversation about what I might or might not want. And most of all I didn't want a scene, because I truly had no idea what he was capable of. Meanwhile Danny was holding up his briefcase.

'Do you want to know what I've got in here?' he asked, eyes widening.

I shook my head.

'Do you want to guess? Come on. Guess. You're such a tease, Sarah. I know you like this stuff really. Let me show you – I've got ropes and gaffer tape and –' He made as if to open it, fingers fiddling with the clasp.

'I don't want to see what's in there, Danny. I want you to go. There's a train coming in a few minutes,' I said. I made an effort to look over towards the train station platforms. He followed my gaze and it gave me the split-second head start and element of surprise that I needed. I got the key in the lock, opened the door and scrambled into the car before he had a chance to grab me – and there was a part of me that was sure he planned to grab me – and engaged the central locking by banging down the little button on the door with my elbow.

Without looking to see what he was doing, I put the key in the ignition and fired up the engine. I'd already made the decision that if Danny stood behind me I would keep going and make him jump out of the way, or hit him if needs be, but he didn't stand behind me. Instead he banged on the windows and the roof of the car with his briefcase, screaming obscenities and trying to kick the door. It seemed to go on forever but it could only have been a few seconds before I was clear of him.

I ignored him and kept on going. Reversing out, I swung round and then headed for the car park exit at a decent speed, but not fast, resisting the temptation to floor it in case I hit someone.

Glancing into the mirror I could see Danny following me, waving his arms and still shouting and swearing. He ran for a few steps but I guess he knew that he was beaten and couldn't catch me up. I prayed that when I got to the station entrance the traffic wouldn't be too heavy so I would be able to pull out before he had the chance to catch me.

At the gates to the station concourse the road was clear. I accelerated away, absolutely certain that I had escaped from something truly dangerous.

Instead of heading into town I turned right towards the bypass that led out of town, thinking that if Danny got a cab and followed me he would be wrong-footed from the start. I took one last look back as I pulled out into the late-morning traffic. Danny was striding back towards the station ticket office.

As I drove back towards town the long way round, I reminded myself that I was safe. Danny didn't know my real name or my address. He did have my mobile phone number and a photograph I had sent him via my anonymous-sounding email address, set up just for the BDSM website, but that was all. In my anxiety, though, I imagined him tracking me down even as I was driving away. I racked my brain, trying to remember what I had told him about myself. He knew I was a writer. Had I told him my pen name?

Irrationally, I didn't want to go home. It felt like, if I did, I would somehow be taking Danny home with me. Instead I pulled into the car park at the back of The Crown and Mitre, where I had been planning to take Danny for lunch. I parked my car over in the far corner, close to the beer garden and children's play area, behind a row of outbuildings, so that anyone taking a casual look around from the entrance wouldn't be able to spot it.

I locked the car and then double-checked that it was locked, imagining Danny coming after me, tracking me from the railway station, breaking into the car and waiting for me in there. There is a real downside sometimes to having an overactive imagination. When I was certain that the car was secure I went inside, trembling, unsteady and acutely conscious of what was going on around me.

I could walk to my house from the pub in under five minutes if I needed to, and thought I might just do that if I felt the need for a drink. Although it was reasonably warm inside I kept on shivering, my teeth chattering. I felt cold right through to the core.

The Crown and Mitre is an old coaching inn, steeped in history, with low beams, flagstone floors and oak-panelled walls. On the ground floor facing the street there is one main central bar, and a fireplace at either end of the room. Beyond that is a modern dining room carved out of what was the old stable block.

In the bar the walls are hung with a bizarre collection of antiques. I've taken family and friends to eat there several times since I moved in, and have often nipped in for Sunday lunch when I couldn't be bothered to cook. They know me there, at least by sight, if not by name.

As I came in through the door the landlord looked up from serving and smiled.

'Well, hello there,' he said. 'In for lunch, are we? Got your favourite on today, steak and ale pudding.'

It was early and there was only a handful of people in the bar. I smiled and nodded to acknowledge the greeting but realised I couldn't speak and that tears weren't far away.

The landlord did a double take. 'You all right, love? You look a bit peaky.'

I nodded. 'I'm fine,' I lied.

'You don't look very fine to me,' he said, coming round to my side of the bar. 'Come and sit down. I've not long lit the fire.'

He made as if to take my arm and it took all my strength not to snatch it away or burst into tears as he shepherded me across the room. When it came right down to it, nothing very much had happened: I had driven away from the danger that I had been in; Danny had gone and I was safe; but that wasn't how it felt. To make matters worse my mind was busy playing out the what-ifs and might-have-beens, and I kept coming back again and again to the fact that I had been stupid to make myself vulnerable in the first place. I had been the one who had squarely put myself in harm's way, and even the fact that I'd gotten away and Danny had presumably left was no consolation.

There are two easy chairs and a sofa by the fire at the far end of the bar. It was the quietest space, away from the main door. The landlord guided me into one of the chairs and said: 'Do you want a drink? You look like you could use one. I could fix you a toddy. You reckon you've got a bug or something? There are some really nasty things going around at the moment.'

Wasn't that the truth?

I thanked him and reassured him that I was okay. I planned to drive home if I could.

'Bit of a funny turn, was it?' he suggested.

'Bit of a shock, that's all,' I said, realising that I had to tell him something and making the effort to smile. He nodded sagely.

'I'll get Lucy to bring you a pot of tea, shall I? Or do you want something stronger?'

I smiled. 'No, tea will be just fine, thank you,' I said.

When Lucy, the barmaid, appeared she had a tray of tea and the menu tucked under her arm. 'His nibs thought you might like to look at this. Said you were a bit shaky.' She slid the menu onto the table alongside the tray. 'Give me a shout when you're ready to order. Sometimes it helps to have a bite to eat if you're feeling a bit woozy.'

I nodded and thanked her for being so kind. While I was waiting for the tea to brew I thought about the bite I had already had. I slipped a hand under my coat and cradled the breast that Danny had bitten. It ached. I wanted to look at it. I wanted to hold it and make it better. When I glanced up I realised that the landlord was looking in my direction. I smiled and picked up the menu, both as a defence and a diversion.

He smiled and nodded as I opened it. I made a show of reading the contents, although I was finding it hard to focus on the words and certainly wasn't taking any of them in. All I wanted to do was sit and think about what had just happened. Think about Danny. Think about our meeting. I ran through it second by second, thanking the god of small mercies that I hadn't suggested he get a taxi to my place and that we go out to lunch from there. It had crossed my mind. I also thanked the same god that when I'd got back from the ticket machine he had got out of the car, and that I had been able to drive away. I just hoped that he had got back on the next train to London and hadn't changed his mind and decided to come up into town to find something to eat. I watched the door from the corner of my eye. Slowly I began to stop shivering as the heat from the fire finally warmed the chill away.

I poured a cup of tea and glanced back at the menu. How could I not have seen the thing with Danny coming? How could I not have seen what he was like? How could I not have recognised that he was unhinged when I'd been speaking to him on the phone? And if I couldn't recognise something so blatant, how could I carry on and trust my instincts when talking to any other Doms in future? It may sound a bit melodramatic, but that was how I felt. I just couldn't believe that Danny had managed to take me in so completely.

'Ready to order now?' asked a female voice, breaking my train of thought. I looked up into the eyes of the barmaid. Her arrival had taken me completely by surprise; I hadn't heard her approaching. I made an effort to compose myself. 'I'm still not sure. Can I have a few more minutes?'

She nodded, although I could see that she was a bit perplexed. 'I always find it hard to make up my mind too,' she said, with a smile. 'Are you sure you're okay? You've not touched your tea. We could call you a cab if you want.'

I glanced down at the tray; I had been holding onto the open menu so long that my arms ached.

'Sorry,' I said, trying to make light of it. 'It's been a bit of a day.'

The girl rolled her eyes. 'I know how that feels. That'll be stone cold and well stewed by now – I'll bring you a fresh pot and that'll give you a chance to decide what you want, all right?'

'Thank you,' I said, as she whisked the tray away.

Glancing up at the clock I was stunned to realise that I had been sitting there for the best part of an hour. Mad, mad, mad – but at least I could be more or less certain that Danny wasn't coming to find me. One of the things I had been trying to remember was whether or not I had told him the name of the place where I'd planned to take him for lunch. The bar had filled up since I'd sat down. That unsettled me; I thought I was being hyper-vigilant, but actually I'd slipped into some sort of shock-induced trance. Interestingly, no one had come and sat near me.

I made an effort to try to pull myself together. I realised I really was hungry and turned my attention back to the menu so that this time when the waitress came back I'd have my order ready.

'Sarah?' I jumped and looked up at the sound of my name, just in time to see Alex heading across the bar towards me. Seeing the anxious expression on his face was the last straw. As Alex got to my table I stood up, and as he took me in his arms I burst into tears. He held me tight up against his chest.

'It's all right. I'm here now. I'm here,' he soothed. 'Where is he? Is he here?' He looked round.

I waved the tears away, mumbling my apologies. 'I'm fine. I'm so sorry. I didn't mean to make a fuss.'

'Where is he?' Alex repeated, looking around the busy bar.

'He's gone,' I said.

Lucy returned with another tray of tea. 'I'll go and get another cup,' she said, as Alex guided me back into the chair and pulled the other one up alongside it.

'So what happened?' he asked earnestly.

I shook my head, feeling my bottom lip tremble; the tremor transferred to my voice. 'It was something, and nothing,' I said, trying hard to make it no big thing. I felt silly, embarrassed, that Danny had tricked me and foolish that I had made Alex drive all this way for nothing, but so very grateful that he had come to my rescue. 'I'm not sure I can explain. Actually, it was awful.'

'You can tell me all about it, but I think you should eat something.' He picked up the menu from the table. 'Do you want lunch? I don't know about you but I'm famished.'

I nodded. 'Me too.'

'Good, okay, let's eat, and then I'll take you home,' he said.

By the time Lucy came back with the extra cup Alex had flicked through the menu and was ready to order. I didn't even bother looking again; I just asked her to bring me the same.

Over lunch I told Alex about the meeting with Danny and tried to convey how threatened I'd felt, how vulnerable and scared. To me it sounded feeble when I said it aloud. I'm not sure that men feel vulnerability in the same way, but Alex listened and nodded. We talked about what Danny's problem might be. We talked about what I had told him and how much of a risk there might be of him showing up.

And we talked about what I should do, if anything. The circumstances made it difficult; after all, I had been expecting a Dom. In defence of his behaviour Danny could so easily say that he had given me exactly what I was expecting and wanted. I'm not sure anyone who wasn't into BDSM would understand the difference between BDSM and the way Danny had behaved.

I imagined the conversation in my head, which went along the lines of: '*So you were expecting that this man, whom you had never met before, might want to spank or hit you?*'

'Yes.'

'*And he did?*'

'Yes.'

'*But not how you wanted to be hit?*'

'That's right.'

'*So how did you want to be hit?*'

'Consensually.'

'*But surely, by agreeing to act out this fantasy you were consenting?*'

It would be a nightmare.

# Chapter Twelve

I can't remember what Alex and I ate for lunch or whether it was good or bad. Alex insisted that I have a brandy and then he paid and drove us back to my house, leaving my car where it was, tucked away in the car park out of sight.

Once we got home, we barely spoke. Instead, Alex took my hand and led me upstairs to the bathroom. He turned on the shower and helped me to undress. He was gentle but insistent, fingers working over the buttons and zip. I didn't resist him. I was exhausted and felt as if I had run a marathon. Everything I took off went straight into the laundry basket.

When I was naked I examined my body in the long bathroom mirror. Almost the whole of my right breast was dark blue where Danny had bitten me. His teeth marks were clearly visible in among the indigo stain of the bruise, and I had livid hand prints around the top of each arm.

If he was shocked, Alex didn't say it. Instead, he turned on the water in the shower. He slipped off his shoes, socks and jacket, left his keys and wallet on the chair and gently led me into the shower and soaped me from head to foot. He worked me over slowly, inch by inch. He was drenched. I can't tell you how touching it was, or how safe and nurtured I felt. The water plastered his hair to his face and his T-shirt and jeans to his body, but he seemed totally unperturbed.

Alex washed my back and my hair, soothing my hurts, easing my tension, whispering soft comforting words as he did his best to wash Danny away. The water and the touch of his fingers were what I needed.

As I began to relax I stretched out towards him, grateful that he had come to my aid, grateful that he had come home with me, grateful for his understanding that what I needed more than anything was to feel clean.

With his hands cradling my face, Alex kissed my closed eyes, and my neck, and my shoulders. He worked his way across my body, planting kisses on each mark on my arms before kissing first my unmarked breast and then the one covered with bruises and teeth marks. His kisses were tender and healing and made me shiver. I groaned softly as he drew a nipple into his mouth, taking the weight of my bitten breast as he sucked gently. The tears that had threatened to flow since Alex started to touch me ran unhindered down my face. I didn't want him to see my tears; I didn't want him to stop touching me.

And against all the odds and every sensible, rational thought, I could feel my body responding to his caresses. I could feel my nipples hardening, feel a dull, hungry ache slowly growing between my legs. I had wondered as I drove away from the station whether I would ever want anything to do with Doms again, but this wasn't coming from any rational place. This was my body, pure and simple. It was a physical reaction, a joyous celebration of the fact that I was still here; I wasn't raped, beaten or dead – possibilities that had crossed my mind more than once while I had been sitting in the pub – I had survived.

Alex's touch was tender and cautious, as if at any moment he expected me to crumble. Finally he slid a hand between my legs; I groaned with pleasure. He kissed me harder, cupping my sex, gently brushing the heel of his hand back and forth over the outer lips, tugging at them, teasing my clitoris but not stimulating it directly. I sighed, letting the sensations build and grow. I could sense his growing excitement and eagerly, hungrily helped him undress, dragging his wet T-shirt up over his back and head and struggling to get his jeans off. We were laughing and kissing, and as Alex stepped out of his underwear I reached down to take his rapidly thickening cock in my hand.

He gasped as my fingers closed around his engorged shaft and began working up and down, making him harder still, making him groan. My slippery soapy hands worked the silky flesh backwards and forwards, finding a rhythm, finding the sweet spot. I ran my fingertips over the sensitive bridge of flesh beneath the head, dragging a nail delicately over the single eye while my other hand teased his balls, brushing and stroking and cupping their weight.

Alex shivered and looked at me so that his gaze locked on mine. Tears all gone, I smiled. I relished the feeling of power as I felt his excitement build. The intensity increased.

'I'm glad you called me,' he said.

'Me too.'

'You need someone to look after you, someone to take you in hand,' he said.

I laughed and renewed my efforts. 'I think you'll find that at the moment it's the other way round, Alex.'

Alex grabbed my wrist and pulled me closer. 'You'll make me come,' he gasped.

'I know,' I said. We were nose to nose now, the water cascading down over the two of us.

Alex kissed me hard. It made my heart do some kind of crazy back flip. I wanted him so much; I wanted to feel him inside me; I wanted to reclaim myself and him from the day. Alex kissed me again and I kissed him back angrily, hungrily, demanding more. Our teeth clashed, our lips locked. He threaded his fingers through my hair and pulled me tight up against him, his mouth working mine, tongue exploring. But I didn't relinquish my hold on his cock; my hand worked frantically to bring him to the edge.

I was torn between this feeling of control and wanting him to fuck me. As he got closer and closer to coming, Alex tightened his grip on my hair and pushed me down onto my knees. I did nothing to resist him. I knew that here and now, with Alex, whatever happened I was safe.

He guided his cock into my mouth, fucking my mouth, dragging me backwards and forwards by my hair, making me cry out, making me gag and whimper, making me tumble into the dark, warm sea that is total submission. At that moment I was his, all other thoughts abandoned. I was gasping, totally absorbed in the moment, totally absorbed taking Alex to the brink, at once – bizarrely – both in control and yet on my knees enacting an ancient act of worship and complete surrender.

The water from the shower was crashing over us, running over my hair and face. I renewed my efforts, sensing that Alex was almost there. He was so close that I knew in another instant there would be no turning back – and at that point Alex pulled out, coming in the same split second, spurting all over my face and in my hair. He let out a throaty growl of pleasure. I could taste the saltiness of his semen as it washed down over my lips; could feel it thick and warm on my face, the pearly droplets clinging to my eyelashes, cheeks and lips.

Before I could wipe it away Alex knelt down in front of me and washed away all traces of his orgasm, and then he kissed me and held me tight up against his chest.

Eventually he helped me to my feet, switched off the shower and wrapped me up in a big white fluffy towel, drying me briskly – and then he took me by the hand and guided me into the bedroom.

'Lie down. On your back,' he said. His tone was cool and strong.

I did as I was told while he watched me. He stood at the end of the bed, towering over me, eyes very slowly working across my bruised body, taking in every last detail. I shivered. I could see the desire in Alex's face and feel my own unfulfilled hunger. I was already turned on and desperate for release.

Alex bent down and pulled my hips to the end of the bed so my feet were on the floor, spreading me wide before sinking to his knees. I knew what was coming and just how much I wanted it. This time there was no working his way down, no slow progress, no nibbling kisses trailing down over my belly. Instead, Alex slid his hands under my buttocks and, lifting me up onto his tongue, began to lap and kiss and suck all those tender, sensitive places – my clitoris, the soft folds of my sex – and while his tongue worked its magic his fingers opened me up, sliding in and out, making me shiver with pleasure.

Alex wasn't gentle, he wasn't tender: he was devouring me whole, driving me further and further into the void, his fingers busy and bold and his tongue licking and thrusting, making me bay with pleasure.

I thrust up to meet his kisses, his tongue, his lips – I was sobbing as he began to suck my swollen clitoris. It was the most amazing, almost overwhelming sensation. I gasped, struggling to hold on as the feelings intensified. He made as if to pull away. It was more than I could bear – I begged him not to stop, and he didn't. And then suddenly, without warning, I started to come and come and come, great waves of intense pleasure rolling through me. My back arched as the sensations ricocheted through my body, hot and red and raw, wave after wave after wave, on and on – I was trembling with delight.

Before I could recover, Alex was up on the bed, between my legs, unrolling a condom. And then he was inside me, driving his renewed cock deep into my wet and eager pussy. He pinned me down, pulling my hands up above my head, pushing me down into the mattress as he drove into me. The feel of him filling my sensitised, quivering sex made me cry out. I relished the feeling of

SARAH K

his hands tight around my wrists, controlling me, holding me.

As he began to move, pressing deeper still, I was stunned as my orgasm rekindled and my body closed tight around him, dragging him deeper and deeper as I thrust upwards, meeting and matching him stroke for stoke. And in that fire, that white-hot fire, all the fear, all the damage that Danny had caused was burnt away and turned to ash, vanishing into the abyss.

And then, at last, we were still. Alex was breathing hard, my breaths were little more than ragged gasping sobs, but we were done. Completely and utterly done. Alex collapsed down onto me, hot and sated, then after a moment rolled over so that he was alongside me and pulled the bedclothes up over us both. He slipped his arm under my shoulders and I rolled over so that we were curled like two spoons, snug under the weight of the duvet, grateful, contented and completely at ease. Alex stroked my hair and my shoulder until I fell into a deep dreamless sleep, safe in his arms, lulled by the sound of his breathing and the beating of his heart.

I woke once, full of panic and faceless, nameless terrors, but Alex was there, murmuring words of comfort and holding me all the closer. I let myself be comforted and curled back into his body. I have no idea what time it was when we woke – late evening, the early hours of the morning? I didn't know or care – but when we did, Alex padded downstairs while I dozed and came back with a tray of tea and buttered toast with poached eggs, which we ate in bed, sitting close to each other, me so grateful, so very grateful, for his comforting presence.

I slept all night in Alex's arms. In that warm, dark space before sleep I thought about the strengths and traits that made a man a Dom. It isn't all tying up, tormenting and nipple clamps; it's about being big enough to care and to nurture and to take charge in other ways, to create and maintain a safe space where someone else can be vulnerable.

As I settled down and let sleep claim me, Alex moved in and kissed my neck.

What woke me the following morning was the sound of a male voice. It was coming from behind the closed door, from out on the landing. It took me a minute or two to get my bearings and put two and two together and remember that Alex had stayed over, and with that came the memories of the previous day and my meeting with Danny. The more I thought about it, the more I realised how lucky I had been to get away as lightly as I had.

I listened to the sounds coming from beyond the closed door, trying to work out what was going on. It sounded as if Alex might be on the phone. I rolled over and picked up my mobile to check the time and was stunned to see that it was almost ten o'clock. Eight o'clock is a lie-in in my life. I couldn't remember sleeping so well or so long for years, but even so, I needed to be getting up and getting on with my day.

Sliding across the bed, I swung my legs over the side and then glanced down. The bruising and bite mark on my breast looked even worse than the day before, and catching sight of it brought the events of the day home with a bang. Up until yesterday's meeting with Danny I had been lucky that every encounter I'd had had gone well and basically been on my terms. My very brief encounter with Danny had come as a complete shock and had truly opened my eyes.

I heard Alex's voice, low and even, the actual words not quite audible through the closed door. I pulled on a robe and opened the bedroom door. Alex was walking up and down the landing, naked except for a towel wrapped around his waist. I could hear the tumble drier rumbling away downstairs, presumably with his T-shirt and jeans in it.

He had the house phone tucked under his chin. His hair was wet from the shower and every bit of me tingled with pleasure as our eyes met. He smiled, but there was something in his expression that unsettled me.

I pulled a face and pointed to the phone, asking the 'what's up?' question without speaking, praying that it wasn't Danny.

'Hi, she's up now,' he said into the phone, and then he held it out towards me, his hand over the mouthpiece. 'I picked it up so it wouldn't wake you.'

'Thank you,' I mouthed. 'Who is it?'

Alex's smile held. 'It's Max,' he said. 'For you.' As if it might be for anyone else.

For a moment everything stood still. I stared at him. 'Max?' I repeated.

Alex nodded. 'I'm just going to get dressed and then I'll fix us some breakfast. Okay?'

I nodded and took the phone from him, my mind racing. My first thought on seeing Alex's face was that somehow Danny had got hold of my home phone number. But Max? I couldn't remember the last time we had spoken. There was something eerie about his timing.

I took a moment or two to compose myself. 'Hello?' I said tentatively.

'Hello, Sarah,' said Max. His voice, so very familiar, was dark and deep and brought a whole raft of memories and emotions flooding back – memories of long nights and fabulous days spent together. We had had a lot of fun. Nights of pleasure and pain, days of companionship and conversation as he had guided my first steps towards submission. His voice made me remember being spanked for the first time, and the first kiss of a whip, the first bite of the cane.

As Alex went back into the bedroom and pulled the door closed behind him, I went into my office and sat down at the desk, feeling unsettled and shaky.

'You rang me before,' I said, remembering the missed call on my mobile.

'That's right, I did. I was rather hoping that you might ring me back. How are you?'

'I'm fine, thank you,' I said, trying to keep my tone neutral as we exchanged pleasantries.

'And who is your friend?' He lingered over the word 'friend', adding a salacious edge.

'Alex,' I said, sounding unexpectedly defensive. 'His name is Alex.'

'And this Alex, he's your new Dom, is he?' Max asked.

I hesitated for a split second. There was no way I intended to explain to Max, of all people, the arrangement that Alex and I had, or why we had come to it. After all, I had only decided not to commit to Alex because I had been so emotionally mangled and uncertain of my own feelings after being involved with Max. But that split second's pause was enough for Max to jump to his own conclusions.

'So that would be a *no* then, would it?' he said with a laugh. 'What is he, a little light diversion or have you got him in to mow the lawn?'

'No,' I snapped. 'I mean, no, it's just complicated.'

Max laughed. 'When we were together it was very straightforward, Sarah. Remember?'

How could I possibly forget?

'I saw that your personal ad is back up on the site,' Max continued conversationally.

'Yes,' I said. 'I thought it was time.'

'So I see. And you didn't think of contacting me first before you put it back up on there?'

'What?' I spluttered. 'Since when do I need your permission?'

'It used to be that you always needed my permission, if you remember. I thought what we had was special.'

There was no denying it: it had been. But in the end I had walked away from the relationship, not because it was over but because I loved him enough to let him go and give him the space to sort out his own very complicated personal life. Walking away from Max had been one of the hardest things I'd ever done in a relationship, but it had been the right thing to do. And although I knew that, it hadn't made it any easier to do or to get over.

'At the very least I thought you might have let me know that you were looking and playing again,' Max said. I thought he sounded hurt and slightly indignant. 'If you didn't feel you could ring, you could have emailed me.'

'What we had is over. I don't need to tell you anything,' I said, my indignation matching his. There was a part of me that wondered exactly who Max thought he was. What did he expect me to do? Spend the rest of my life pining for him? Join a convent? Creep back to vanilla relationships because there would never be anyone quite like him?

'I know that.' Max laughed. 'And I know that voice. I can imagine the look on your face, Sarah. I was just a bit surprised to see you on the site, that's all. I suppose I shouldn't have been, but I was.' He paused. 'I wanted to make sure that you were okay and I wanted to let you know that I've missed you, Sarah. I've missed you a lot.'

I closed my eyes, angry with him for calling, angry with myself for being so affected by the sound of his voice. Wasn't it true that I had missed him too? How many nights had I cried myself to sleep persuading myself that ringing him would only bring me more hurt? I had had to wean myself off him and let myself heal. I said nothing.

His voice dropped to a low, conspiratorial purr. 'After everything we've shared, I thought you might have the good grace to give me first refusal.'

The words shook me out of my little trip down memory lane. I nearly choked. 'You've got a nerve, Max. First refusal? What exactly is that supposed to mean?'

'That life changes, and what we had was good. You know that. I don't have to persuade you that what we had was special. It really hurt me when you left, Sarah. I understand why you did and I respect you for it, but I still think about you every day. Things are different now. I've sorted a lot of things out. I'm in Rome at the moment but I'm going to be back in the UK next week. We should meet up. Talk. See if we can work it out.'

'There's nothing to work out,' I said.

'Really? In that case, come and have a drink with me just for old times' sake.'

'Because?'

'Because we still have things we need to say, Sarah. Things we need to do. And maybe things we need to have another chance at. Don't you feel that too?'

I sat very still. I was torn. Max had broken my heart, or at least my pulling away from him had, but then I thought about Alex. After the night before I had made up my mind that I was a fool not to trust my instincts about him. He deserved better than this.

My silence was Max's cue. 'Lots of things have changed in my life, Sarah, but I don't want to talk about it over the phone. Let's meet. I'll book us into a hotel —'

'That's a bit presumptuous, isn't it? I'm not sure —' I began, intending to go on to say 'that there's any point', but Max cut me short.

'I don't need you to be sure. I just need you to say yes. Please, Sarah. Look, don't say anything now. Think about it. I'll email you the details.' And with that, Max hung up.

I sat cradling the phone in my hand, split between outrage at his arrogant assumptions that I would come running when he called and the dull ache in my heart that walking away from him had left me with. I have always been of the opinion that it is a mistake to go back to anything. I was cross with myself for not telling him that I'd moved on, that I was over him, that it had been good but I had better things on the horizon. The combination of Max and Danny was almost too much. I felt as if everything was shifting.

I went downstairs, still in my robe. Alex was in the kitchen making tea. There was toast and marmalade on the table and flowers from the garden in a milk jug.

'Morning,' he said. His hair was ruffled now, damp and curling. He was wearing his jeans and T-shirt and was padding barefoot around my kitchen. He smiled at me and my heart fluttered.

'Okay?' he asked.

I nodded.

Alex's dominance was a subtler thing than Max's, but it was always there in the dynamic between us. He made me feel feminine and precious, and the erotic charge that gave me was magical. He made me feel safe and cared for. He was strong, a real alpha male, and yet he brought with him a blend of vanilla and BDSM that I suspected was right for me.

I sat down at the kitchen table. Alex carried on getting breakfast. Nothing in his body language suggested that he was in the slightest bit rattled or wrong-footed by Max's phone call. I waited, wondering if he would say something, but he didn't, and finally, unable to bear it any longer, I cracked first. 'I wasn't expecting Max to ring,' I said.

Alex nodded. 'I wondered if maybe you'd called him yesterday when you were having the problem with what's his name.'

I stared at him. 'Are you serious?' I said. Alex had been the person I'd thought of immediately; ringing Max hadn't even crossed my mind.

'Yes, why not? You were in a hole. If I thought that he was closer than me I'd have rung him myself.'

I shook my head. 'It didn't occur to me to ring him, Alex. Max and I split up ages ago now. I told you –'

'You did. You told me that you walked away from something that was special and that you wanted. And if things had been different you'd probably still be with him now, wouldn't you?'

He was right. I nodded.

'And now I get the impression from Max that things have changed.'

'You spoke to him?' I asked in amazement.

Alex nodded. 'A little bit. He sounds like a nice guy.'

'He is. He wants to see me again,' I said. There was no room for lies between us.

'Okay,' said Alex, with a nod.

'What do you mean, "okay"?' I asked incredulously.

He pulled out a chair and sat down next to me. 'You should go,' he said. 'You have to go.'

'I *have* to go? What is this, an order?'

He laughed and shook his head. 'No, of course not. But if you don't go then whether we're together or not you'll always regret it. Might-have-beens have a way of coming back to haunt you.'

'You mean it, don't you?' I said.

Alex nodded, tracing a finger across the back of my hand. 'I want to be your Dom, Sarah. More than that, I want to be with you. But I'm not anyone's also-ran. I want you to be with me because I'm your first choice, not a this'll-do-because-I-can't-have-what-I-really-want. You need to decide what it is you want. Until you sort this out with Max, I don't think you'll be able to do that.'

'There isn't anything to sort out,' I said.

Alex shrugged. 'Then there's nothing for me to worry about, is there?' he said, passing me a mug of tea. 'How do you fancy a drive out to pick up your dress for the party? We could have something to eat while we're there. Or maybe we could drive down to the coast. Cash owes us lunch, remember?'

I looked at him. 'How can you be so calm?'

Alex grinned. 'I've always believed that what's mine will come to me – eventually,' he said. 'It might take a while, but you're worth the wait.'

I stared at him. I wished I was as confident as he was.

'So, what do you fancy? Dress, beach or something else?' he said, eyes still bright with amusement.

'Aren't you supposed to tell me?'

He laughed. 'Aren't you supposed to tell me, *Sir*,' he added.

I was considering his suggestions when a thought struck me. 'I can't try the dress on,' I said. 'Not with these bruises.' The last time I'd been to the dress shop the assistant had insisted on helping me into the dress, and I couldn't see it would be any different this time. The dress had narrow straps and no sleeves, and I could just imagine the woman suggesting I try it without the jacket to see how the alterations had turned out – whichever way I looked at it, keeping the bruises hidden was going to be a problem.

'You don't have to try it on,'

'I want to make sure it fits.'

Alex nodded. 'Stand up and take off your robe,' he said, waving me to my feet.

I thought he was going to take a look at the bruises, but I was wrong.

'Now,' he snapped.

Slowly I got to my feet and did as I was told, feeling horribly self-conscious in the harsh mid-morning light. I hadn't showered. I hadn't done my hair or brushed my teeth. The robe dropped to the floor. I was naked underneath.

Alex smiled. 'Good girl. Put your hands on top of your head,' he said. His tone was dark now, more intense. He got to his feet and walked around me, inspecting me, his eyes as invasive as any touch. His gaze lingered my arms and my breast, taking in the details of the bruises and the bite.

'I was stupid,' I said, feeling my colour rising.

'Did I say you could speak?' Alex asked.

I shook my head. In the space of a few seconds, we had slipped into the intense other world of BDSM, both moving by an unspoken but mutual agreement into role.

Alex took one of the cotton napkins from the table and, folding it, tied it tight over my eyes. The darkness was welcome.

'You weren't stupid,' he said. 'You weren't to know what Danny was like. People like him put a lot of effort into trying to seem like everyone else. You were misguided in meeting him from the train and offering to drive him, but he would have been crazy wherever you met him. And you got yourself out of it.'

Only just, I thought. Meeting Danny had made me rethink a lot of things.

As Alex spoke he took me by the shoulders and guided me through the kitchen door into the inner hallway. When we reached the foot of the stairs he stopped me and turned me around so that I was facing the treads.

'Stand still,' he said. I felt him slip past me and heard him climb the stairs and then, a few seconds later, return. Taking my hands, he buckled on leather cuffs and secured them at the wrist to something he must have slung over the balcony or between the bannisters above us.

He tied me tightly, pulling my hands up above my head so that I was at full stretch. 'There,' Alex said, apparently to himself. 'You look just fine to me. I'm going to beat you and then we're going to go out, bruises or no bruises. Do you understand?'

'Yes, Sir,' I said.

'That's good.' Alex ran his hands over my body – my back, my hips, over my waist and breasts – calming me, soothing me, settling me for whatever was coming next.

Something happens when I am tied, and feeling safe. I can feel myself slipping into a trance-like state that accompanies submission. It is almost like meditation. I am calm. The chatter in my head slowly dies away and I turn inwards. It is a compliant stillness that is oddly peaceful.

Alex trailed something down over my shoulder and back. I shivered. I guessed exactly what it was: the deceptively soft feathery fronds of a suede flogger.

'I bought you a little treat,' he said. 'Let's road test it, shall we?'

'Did you bring that with you when you were on your way to rescue me?' I asked incredulously, heedless of the no-talking rule.

Alex laughed. 'I'd like you to think I was that single-minded and heartless, but no, I met the postman on my way to the car. I had to sign for it.'

Now it was me who laughed, breaking the moment.

'Do you want me to gag you?' he asked. I could hear the amusement in his voice, but also something else, something that was wresting back control.

'No, Sir,' I said.

'Because I can.'

'No, Sir, please don't.'

'Better,' he said. 'Much better.' The fronds of the flogger trickled down my back again, like a caress or the slightest breath of air. I shivered.

'Tell me that you want this, Sarah,' he said. 'Tell me that you need this.' The suede strips ran down my spine again. 'Ask me to beat you.'

'I need this,' I said. I shivered again, the emotion and expectation resonating in my voice.

'You have to ask me. I want you to beg me to flog you,' said Alex, leaning in close so that he was practically whispering in my ear. 'Say it.'

'Please, Sir, flog me,' I whispered.

'Not good enough. Say it again,' said Alex, his voice stronger now.

'Please, Sir, flog me,' I repeated, louder this time.

'Not loud enough,' he said, sounding almost jubilant.

'Please, Sir, flog me!' I cried, almost shouting this time. The words were barely out of my mouth when the first blow exploded across my back, a fusillade of tiny crackling, stinging blows. I gasped. He was right: this was what I needed. I cried out, pulling hard against my bonds. Here, in this bizarre hinterland of pain and surrender, I knew I could find myself, put myself back together; here, in pain, I could find a place that was impossible to access any other way, and oddly it was here that I felt safest and most true to who I am.

While it definitely stung, the blow wasn't hard.

'Count,' said Alex. 'Let me hear you.'

'One,' I said, my voice thick with emotion.

'Louder,' he said.

'One,' I repeated, louder as he demanded.

'Good girl.'

The second blow was a little harder, but not much. It seemed like Alex was taking it steady, feeling his way, taking me there step by tiny step to ensure that after my run-in with Danny I wasn't overwhelmed or distressed.

'Two,' I said in a firm, clear voice.

The third stroke was more intense, the fronds spreading across my shoulders in a tingling arc, still not hard but enough to make me suck the air in between my teeth as the flogger hit home. 'Three,' I said, as the heat rolled through me.

'I want you,' Alex murmured, as he struck me again. 'I want to love you and keep you safe. I want to be the one who does this to you, for always, Sarah. I want to be with you.'

The words were compelling and unexpected. They brought tears to my eyes.

'Four,' I gasped. This time he hit me hard. The fronds were fire and ice, making my skin sing.

'But you have to be sure.'

'Five.'

'I want you to be certain.'

Six, and Alex was finding his form and hitting his stride. The sensations rolled through me: waves of heat, waves of biting pain. I cried out, straining against the ties.

'And there is only one way.'

Seven, and all of me, every last shred of me, was alight.

Eight, and I was gasping for breath, my fists curled tight around the ties, the count all but forgotten as Alex hit me again. It stung so much that this time I shrieked, caught up in the moment. With pain all there is is the now, the moment. Nothing else matters.

'Nine.' And I am crying now, tears rolling down my face. I have cried more in the last twelve hours than I have in weeks. I know the safe word, I can stop this at any time, but I crave the release that the pain is bringing me.

'Ten.' And I am sobbing.

There is something cleansing and healing in the pain. I feel as if I am riding a great wave of emotion and sensation that is somehow restoring me.

'Eleven.' The blow seems less painful, but perhaps it's because my senses are already overloaded. I'm a mess, straining and twisting on the restraints, calling out, begging, and all the while the safe word hangs between us, within easy reach but not the solution I crave.

'Twelve.' And the word is just a noise, an abstraction, and the blow is a sensation a long way from where I am.

'Thirteen. Fourteen.' I am saying the words, marking the moments, but without feeling connected to them. Fifteen, sixteen, and I feel as if I am flying, fuelled by the pain and the endorphin rush it brings with it.

Finally, at twenty, Alex drops the flogger on the stairs, takes off the blindfold and unties my hands. My knees buckle. He kisses my neck and shoulders as he takes my weight. As I regain control he pushes me down onto the stairs so that I am taking my weight on my hands. He is opening my legs wide, touching me, exploring me, while the heat and tingling sensations from the flogging glow red hot across my back and shoulders.

He is stroking me now, finding all those places that make me mewl with pleasure – my clitoris, my g-spot – stroking, circling and pressing. And I move against him, impaling myself on his fingers.

As I get more and more aroused I hear Alex groan with pleasure and unzip his fly. He is slipping off his clothes, but I don't look back. I'm still caught up in the strange otherness that submission creates in me. Seconds later I feel his cock brushing against my inner thighs, hard and hungry, begging for entry.

I reach back to guide him inside me – Alex is rock hard – and I dip my pelvis to give him greater access, encouraging him deeper. His hands catch hold of my hips and he is no sooner inside me than he finds his rhythm, pressing in and out of my wet and eager body.

Desperate for release, I slide my hand back between my legs, seeking out the swollen bud of my clitoris.

'What do you think you're doing?' growls Alex.

'Please, Sir,' I beg. 'I need to come.'

He laughs, deep and throaty and raw. 'I can see that.'

My fingers move lower, working tentatively at the junction where our bodies meet. I graze a fingernail along the seam between his balls. Alex gasps and pushes deeper, the thrust an instinctive reaction, and then our fingers join forces, touching, exploring. As we move together, pushing on and on towards our goal, I am struck by the heady scent of arousal, the rich perfume of our bodies, of sex, of heat and desire.

As Alex slides in and out of me I trace his progress with my fingers. He strokes and presses my clitoris. We are locked in a race towards release. His touch is deft and knowing – mine too. It feels as if we are in intimate competition to bring the other home, and I fear that I am losing. Alex has the most compelling, intuitive touch. I can feel myself sliding over the brink, but I guess from his breathing that Alex isn't far behind. I'm stunned that he can hold on. He circles, he caresses. I am crying out with pleasure now, sobbing, whimpering, the pain of the flogging a distant memory. And then suddenly I'm there; I'm lost. I am falling, plummeting into the abyss, my sex tightening around his shaft, dragging him after me.

I hear Alex gasp. He is so close behind. I feel his cock spasm, hear the change in his breathing and we are both there, chasing each other on and on to the end. I'm afraid that I might fall forwards onto the stairs, my knees are so trembling and soft, but Alex puts a hand out to steady us as he thrusts again, milking those last fleeting sensations. I move with him, not wanting to miss the last sparks flickering through me. And then we are still, sweating, breathing frantically. I can hear my pulse thundering in my ears.

Alex nuzzles into my neck and then slides out of me. 'More tea?' he gasps, with laughter in his voice.

I look back over my shoulder and we are both laughing now; the sounds are warm and childlike. He takes me in his arms and kisses me hard. I relish the sensation and relish his warmth.

He takes my hand and leads me upstairs. 'Get back into bed,' he says, as we get to the bedroom door. 'We can go out for lunch later.'

I don't resist.

# Chapter Thirteen

Less than a week later I was standing all alone outside Victoria Station, dressed to kill in red patent high heels, a little black dress that clung to every curve which I had last worn to another writer's swanky launch party, my Burberry mac, seamed stockings and considerably more make-up than I'd normally wear outside of a fancy-dress party.

I felt like a hooker, although my reflection reminded me that I was in fact a smart, if slightly overdressed, woman in her mid-forties, sporting a new hairdo and quite a lot of lipstick.

As per Max's very explicit instructions, I wasn't wearing any underwear, I was completely shaved and I was feeling the cold. It is one thing to be knickerless when you're with your Dom; quite another entirely when wandering around London trying to find a taxi in the rain – and it *was* raining, hard. A biting wind whipped along the pavement, making it feel colder still. I'd done this kind of thing lots of times before when meeting Max, dressed up or undressed up, depending on his instructions, waiting for our eyes to meet across some public space, all ready for him. And under the right circumstances, it has a real erotic charge and builds a sense of expectation. Today, it was just making me feel grumpy.

The queue for the taxis was moving at a crawl. I was standing at the rank, at the end of the queue, shuffling forwards an inch at a time, wondering what exactly I was doing there. Wondering, in fact, whether I should be there at all. I'd been having the same thoughts and doubts on the train all the way into town.

I'm not denying that there was a part of me that was eager to see Max again. In the time since we split up I had missed him and often wondered how he was or where he was and if he ever thought about me, but in reality I had also come a long way since we were together. I had a clearer idea of what it was I wanted and I was afraid that by seeing Max I might lose that clarity and risk opening the wounds that it had taken me so long to recover from.

True to his word, Max had sent me an email immediately after we had spoken on the phone, which arrived while Alex and I were downstairs. The tone had been as cool, clipped and formal as anything Max had ever sent to me. He invited me to spend the weekend with him in London in a very nice hotel. He set out exactly what I should wear, what I should bring and even suggested which train I should catch. Classic Max. I wouldn't have been at all surprised if he had sent me the rail tickets for the trip – something he'd done before.

Reading his email, I realised I'd forgotten quite how controlling Max was, and also how I had come to accept and even relish the sense of free fall that being with him gave me. When we were together I didn't have to think for myself, order a meal or book a room, because he would do it all. He saw it as an integral part of his role as my Dom and Master. Stepping into his world and relinquishing all control had been addictive.

As someone who is naturally independent, it had taken me a while to adjust to the reality of submission but – because I didn't live with him – I quite enjoyed the time we spent together when I was completely without responsibility. It wasn't that he didn't respect me or realise that I was perfectly capable of making up my own mind and looking after myself, but rather that, when we were together and in role, he enjoyed treating me like an expensive, well-loved and much-treasured pet.

Initially I had to learn that it was okay to let go and to trust that he would take care of me. But the invitation to join him in London was different. We weren't a couple any more, and his assumptions that we could just pick up where we had left off annoyed me.

In my reply to his email I'd taken the same formal tone and expressed my regret that under no circumstances would I be spending the weekend with him. He couldn't assume after all this time that he had that kind of control over me, nor that I would just drop everything and do his bidding. Although I was very happy to meet up with him and talk, I wouldn't be staying. No way.

'Let's wait and see, shall we? I'm booking a room whether you plan to stay or not,' his next email read. 'I want to be able to spend some time with you and talk to you in private.'

I had no problem with that.

And then he had written: 'Bring an overnight bag in case you change your mind,' which made me laugh. You had to give him credit for trying.

I had pointedly done no such thing. So why had I complied with the rest of his requests: the clothes, the current knickerless state? The same thought kept running through my head as I waited for a cab. Old habits? A secret longing to take up where we had left off?

The answer had to be yes, because annoyed or not there was a part of me, the romantic part, that wondered if – maybe even hoped – I would walk in, see him, be totally overwhelmed and find myself swept up in his strong arms and carried away to some sort of mythical happy-ever-after.

It wasn't likely, but I write romance – I'm almost contractually obliged to think in terms of grand passions and the big finish. All the way up to London I was concerned about whether I was doing the right thing or making a terrible mistake, and the uncertainty wasn't helping my mood.

The queue for the taxi was barely moving. My feet were frozen. There were several groups of tourists ahead of me. The couple immediately in front of me were having a domestic. I was shivering. This was madness. I heard my phone ping to announce an incoming message and, grateful for the distraction and wondering if it was from Max, I pulled it out of my handbag and opened it up. It was from Alex and read:

I hope you have a good time. I am torn between hoping that you find what you're looking for and hoping that you don't. Whatever happens, you know that I wish you well. Let me know if I need to put my ad back on the website. Love A x

The words made my eyes well up with tears. What the hell was I doing? Alex deserved so much more than this.

I glanced down at my ridiculous shoes and made a decision. I abandoned the idea of queuing for a cab and headed for the Tube station instead; in less than fifteen minutes I was on Oxford Street, hitting the shops that were still open. There was something I really needed to do before I met Max. Something that would give me the distance and the control I needed. Something that would level the playing field.

'You're late,' Max said, as I walked up to the table. He was sitting in the lobby of the hotel at a table in an alcove that was facing the door. We had agreed to meet for a drink. And he was right, I was late. Very late. I slipped off my coat and he looked me up and down, his eyes alight with a mixture of amusement and surprise.

'I see you decided to ignore my instructions,' he said, steepling his fingers in front of his lips in a gesture I had completely forgotten.

I smiled and pulled out a chair. 'Lovely to see you too, Max,' I said. 'I did text you to say that I'd been held up.'

He got to his feet and kissed me on both cheeks, leaning in close so that he could whisper: 'I'm going to punish you for this, you know? Or is that exactly what you're hoping for?'

I pulled away and raised my eyebrows. 'For texting you or for getting held up?'

He laughed. 'For everything. You should have called me and let me know where you were.'

'The battery in my phone is almost dead,' I said.

'You won't need it now,' he said, and then, glancing down at the scrum of carrier bags that I had set down on the floor by the table, he added: 'If you wanted to go shopping we could have gone together. Tomorrow.'

I laughed. 'Tomorrow?'

He nodded.

'I won't be here tomorrow, Max. I've already told you that.'

'We'll see …' He waved the waiter over.

My detour to Oxford Street had involved finding a whole new outfit and changing the balance of power. I was now dressed in a really nice chocolate-brown suit and new boots – and I had my knickers on. I was a lot warmer and far more comfortable than I had been earlier, and I guessed from Max's expression that I had completely wrong-footed him. My other outfit, the one he had instructed me to wear, was now neatly folded up and tucked inside one of the shopping bags at my feet, along with the red killer heels.

'Drink?' Max asked.

I nodded. 'Oh yes, please. I'd love a cup of tea. I'm frozen,' I said, rubbing my hands together. 'It's really cold out there today.'

He smiled. We both knew he didn't mean that kind of drink. 'I told you to take a taxi.'

'I did, eventually,' I said casually.

Max looked me over and then checked his watch.

'Expecting someone else?' I joked.

'No, actually I was calculating exactly what your punishment should be: lateness, incorrect dress, forgetting to call me Sir. I've got plenty to be going on with.' He leaned in closer. 'Tell me, Sarah, what is it that you've missed the most?'

A waiter arrived before I could reply. Max picked up one of the menus, which had been sitting on the table between us. The waiter looked enquiringly in my direction, but before I could speak Max ordered a drink and then went on to order dinner for both of us. I smiled at him as he told the man what we wanted.

'Old habits die hard,' I said, as the waiter wrote down the order. Max deciding what I ate when we were together had always been one of the cornerstones of our relationship.

'Apparently not in every case,' said Max archly, giving me a stern look. I assumed that he was suggesting that without his guidance I had gone feral.

While Max was sorting out the finer points of our meal, I took the opportunity to give him the once over. It seemed like an age since I'd last seen him. He was looking good; he was tanned and had lost weight since we were in Paris. His hair was cut differently, which made him look younger. But some things hadn't changed. Max still had the same air of reserve and quiet self-assurance that had attracted me to him in the first place, and which I had always found both exciting and compelling.

As I was looking at him he glanced up at me under heavy brows and, for a moment, as our eyes met, he held my gaze. I felt my heart do that little back-flippy thing that hearts do. I knew how he worked; I'd been here many times before. Max didn't smile, he just looked into me.

When we were together as Dom and sub, this little trick of his, this cool, appraising, predatory stare, would turn me to jelly. Today, as our eyes met, I smiled and he was the one who looked away first.

People always treated Max as if he were somebody. The waiter did it as Max turned his attention back to the food. The man was deferential and wore an expression that suggested he felt he should know who Max was, but couldn't quite place him. I watched Max's face. While he was always polite, he also always assumed that people would treat him well and with deference, and as a result they inevitably did.

Settling now, I contemplated exactly what I was doing there. When I had first walked into the hotel and spotted Max sitting in the corner of the lounge waiting for me, for a moment I had thought about turning around and leaving, rather than risk stirring up all those emotions that had been there before. My heart had ached a little when our eyes met, and then he had smiled as I made my way over to him. But I hadn't had some big moment of revelation when I realised that I had made a terrible mistake in leaving him. Instead, as I sat there opposite him, Max felt like someone I had known a long, long time ago – an old friend, a good friend, but not someone I still loved. By choosing a fabulous famous hotel to eat and stay in, Max was making a statement about the kind of man he was and what he could offer me. He seemed to have forgotten that I already knew. He didn't need to impress me.

'Did you bring the outfit I asked you to wear?' he asked, when the waiter left.

Without thinking, I glanced down briefly at the shopping bags.

Max laughed. 'I might have guessed. So, not completely disobedient after all, then?' he said. 'Or are you keeping your options open?' When I didn't reply he said: 'So, how have you been?'

I nodded. 'Fine, thank you,' I said.

He tipped his head to one side. 'What sort of answer is that?'

And without really understanding why, I found myself trying hard not to let my bottom lip tremble or my eyes fill with tears.

'I'm okay,' I said, struggling to keep the tremor out of my voice. 'Busy. I've got a new book out next month. And work, well, you know – always something to do.' I could feel him watching me, but I made the effort to keep up the chatter until the moment of panic and pain had passed. I pressed on talking about real life, the life I led away from BDSM and relationships, until the waiter arrived with our drinks and there was a natural pause in the conversation.

'So, you haven't missed me at all then?' Max asked, once the waiter had retreated.

By now I was recovered and strong enough to say: 'Of course I have. I missed you for months, Max. I thought about you every day. But if you're asking me if I regret walking away from what we had, then no, I don't. You needed the space and time to sort things out, and I –'

He held up a hand, stemming the flow of words. 'I understand, Sarah. I know why you did it. I just wanted to know if you ever thought you were wrong. Whether you regretted it.'

I took a breath to answer him, but Max continued. 'Look, why don't we finish our drinks and take dinner up in my room? We'll have a lot more privacy up there.' He lifted a hand to attract the waiter's attention.

I looked at Max and laughed. 'So that you can get my clothes off?'

Max shrugged, eyes bright with humour. 'Well, the thought had crossed my mind. Don't tell me you hadn't had the same thought,' he said, and then he grinned. 'I can't believe you showed up dressed like that, Sarah.' And with that, any lingering tension that had hung between us evaporated. 'The suit, the boots ...' He made a gesture to encompass the outfit. 'You might as well have worn a suit of armour. I gave you specific instructions. You know the rules.'

'Which I ignored.'

'You don't say,' he said.

'You're forgetting: I'm not your subbie any more, Max.'

He leaned in closer. 'But we both know that could change, don't we? Tell me that you don't miss submission.'

'I didn't say I didn't.'

'So what's stopping you? Why resist? We could start over. What we had was good, you know that.'

I smiled. I did know that, but I also knew something else about what we had – that Max had kept parts of his life neatly hidden and compartmentalised, and that the first thing I had known about his other life was when his resident, albeit ex, partner had turned up in Paris with their daughter in tow.

'How is Abby?' I asked, stirring my tea.

Max narrowed his eyes. 'Oh, touché,' he said, miming a flinch. 'She is good. Actually, she is better than good. She and Ellie moved back into their own place a few months ago. Her house is all sorted out after the water leak and she's found herself another job. Only part time at the moment, but she is really enjoying it, and her parents are covering the childcare, so I'm seeing less of them both, but in some ways I think that is better for us. We talk on the phone and when she drops Ellie off. She seems really well and happy.'

I waited, sensing that there was more, and I was right.

'And she is seeing someone. I've met him a couple of times; he seems like a really nice guy. I thought I should meet him if he is going to be part of my daughter's life.'

I nodded.

'So the two of them are doing just fine,' he added.

'Is that why you rang me?' I asked, watching his face.

'Yes and no. I didn't want to get in touch until I was certain that Abby was okay. But the truth is I missed you, Sarah; you must know that. Every single day. And okay, you did the right thing, and I admire you for it, but it was still bloody painful. For both of us. And then I went online and saw your ad on the website, and it seemed like fate.'

'Fate?'

Max nodded. 'You just said that you missed me too. So here we are, just like old times. Things back to how they were, how they should be – all except for that ridiculous outfit,' said Max. 'You know what I want, Sarah. I want us to start over. We were good together.'

I stared at him. He was right, but things had changed. More truthfully, *I* had changed, and I now had a far clearer idea of what I wanted and I told him so.

'We've talked about this before: vanilla and BDSM together don't work. You know that. You can have one or the other, but not both.'

'But I want both,' I said.

'You always were greedy,' Max laughed.

'I've met other people, other Doms, who want the same thing as I do,' I snapped, and in spite of my best efforts I knew I sounded defensive and slightly petulant.

He snorted. 'Really? So why are you here tonight if you have already found what you want with someone else?'

Max's words hit a real nerve. I paused and then, as calmly as I could, said: 'Because I wanted to see you.'

That much was true; I had been curious to see how he was and whether that grand passion I had felt before was still there. I had known from the moment our eyes met that it had gone, but I was still glad that I'd come. Alex had been right: without meeting Max again, I would never have known that it was well and truly dead.

But that wasn't Max's view on it. 'When it comes right down to it, Sarah, you know that I'm right. You're here because you miss what we had – you miss me and, whether you have admitted it to yourself or not, you want to come back.' He took a sip of wine from the glass on the table between us. 'Why fight it?'

I stared at him, astounded by his assumptions, and laughed. 'You are such an arrogant bastard,' I said.

'I agree. Anyway,' he continued, as if I hadn't spoken, 'whatever you've been doing over the last few months we can chalk up to experience. You can tell me all about it later.' He took a room key out of his jacket pocket and slid it across the table. 'Go upstairs and get changed. I'm assuming you did bring a more suitable outfit with you.' This time it was he who glanced at the shopping. 'Or did you buy something special just for me?'

There was something in his tone and his assumption that nothing I had done or no one I had met since leaving him could possibly be more important or significant than him that infuriated me. I didn't move. The key lay between us.

He looked at me. 'What is it?' he said. 'I assumed from the fact that you came to meet me that you want the same things that I want.'

'Well, that is a big assumption, Max. I said I'd come and meet you so that we could talk.'

He laughed. 'Oh come on, Sarah. We know each other better than that. You didn't think that we would end up playing?'

I felt another flicker of outrage. Of course it had crossed my mind. Hadn't I been weighing up the possibilities and probabilities since getting his email? What galled me was his presumption that there was no doubt I'd go straight back to what we had.

He leaned closer. 'What's changed?' he asked, his tone not cool but inquisitive.

'Everything,' I replied quietly.

'So, are you saying that on this quest to find both you *have* met someone?'

I hesitated for a split second. 'I've met a lot of people since we split up.'

Max raised his eyebrows. 'That isn't what I asked you, Sarah, and you know it. I meant someone special, someone who means that instead of coming here today dressed as I instructed you came here dressed like *that*.' He waved a hand in my direction.

I laughed. 'Do I look that bad?'

'No, of course not, you look beautiful. But you know exactly what I mean.'

He watched my face as if he might be able to find the answers there, and of course he could.

'His name is Alex,' I said.

Max nodded. 'Alex. I spoke to him.'

Of course he had. His expression softened. 'I thought you'd come back to me, but it looks as if you came here to say goodbye.'

I stared at Max for a moment and realised that he was right. I didn't want him back. And I needed to explain why.

The waiter came to tell us that our table was ready. Dinner came and went. We talked on and on for hours. I didn't intend to tell Max about my deal with Alex, nor why I'd struck it. I didn't mean to tell him about my encounter with Danny and how shaken it had left me, nor about how grateful I had been that Alex had come to my rescue. I didn't mean to tell Max about how much it had meant to lie curled up in Alex's arms afterwards, nor anything about how I truly believed that with him I had found a way to mix vanilla and the compelling kink of BDSM. I didn't mean to tell him that I thought I had finally found a man I could truly love. But I did.

We talked about what I wanted and what I needed, and he reminded me of what it was that he could offer, and the things that made what we had special. We talked about the time we had had together and, prompted by him, I remembered little details I'd forgotten. Even as we were laughing and talking, we both knew that it was finally over, but it was good to tie up all the ragged painful ends of what had been something good.

Finally, when they brought our coffee, it was Max not me who brought the conversation back to Alex and how much he meant to me.

'So, this thing with Alex, it's serious then?' he asked.

I considered the idea for a moment and then I nodded. I just hadn't realised quite how serious it was until that moment.

Max smiled sadly. 'I was hoping we might start over, but it's too late, isn't it?'

I nodded.

He smiled. 'It was fun.' Max glanced at his watch. 'What time did you say your train was?'

I looked up from the table. The restaurant was almost empty. I had no idea we'd been sitting there for so long. I glanced at my watch, feeling for all the world like Cinderella just before the clock struck twelve.

The sight of the time jolted me back to reality. 'I really have to go,' I said, hastily getting to my feet. It wasn't just my train I was afraid of missing.

'You could stay,' Max said, and for a moment our eyes met, but whatever it was he saw in my face made him smile sadly. 'Okay, forget I said that. Why don't you at least let me sort out a cab for you?' He waved to the waiter as I anxiously gathered my possessions. While someone went to find my coat and another went to find me a taxi, I was filled with a growing sense of dread.

I realised that I hadn't replied to Alex's text and wondered how long it would take for him to decide that waiting was futile. What if I was too late? What if, because he hadn't heard from me, Alex had already put his profile back up? It was irrational, but the sense of anxiety pressed down on me, along with a pile of other thoughts ...

How would I feel if it had been him, not me, en route to spend an evening with an old flame? I certainly wouldn't have taken it so calmly. Alex had been at home and on holiday for the last two weeks. We had spent much of it together. He asked nothing from me, no commitment, no promises, just the simple pleasure of being together, sharing a desire to explore BDSM together. Sometimes when we were together I was kneeling on the floor beside the sofa in a leather collar and cuffs; sometimes I was curled up on the sofa beside him sharing a pizza. Max was wrong; it was possible to have both if you chose the right person. And I knew, without a shadow of a doubt, that Alex was the right person.

Max caught my hand. 'Take care,' he said, and kissed my cheek. The kiss was as chaste as something you'd expect from a maiden aunt. 'And be happy, Sarah. Alex is a lucky man. If you ever change your mind –'

I laughed. 'I won't,' I said, and hugged him tightly. 'I hope you find what you're looking for, Max,' I said, eyes bright with tears.

'I thought I had,' he said.

I clambered into the taxi, not looking back, praying that I wouldn't miss my train and not wanting to think about what would happen if I did, nor where I would stay. As the taxi pulled away from the hotel I took my phone out of my bag and tapped in Alex's number; the battery's critical warning icon flashed up on the screen, the phone rang twice and then it died in my hand.

I stared at it, wondering what the hell Alex would think. Would he think I was ringing to tell him it was over? Would the two rings make him think I couldn't find the words or the courage to tell him? Would he try to ring me back only to find that he couldn't get through? Two rings were worse than no rings at all.

At the station I had to run, but I made the train with just seconds to spare.

The train journey home seemed to take forever. As it was the last train of the day, it stopped at every junction, halt and two-horse town all the way home. It was also packed with people on their way home from parties, late-night revellers, drunks and those coming home from working late shifts in the City. I stood for the first half of the journey, thinking about Alex, thinking about the things that Max had said.

The carriages slowly emptied as the train got closer and closer to home. I was wishing every mile gone.

The only real upside was that – wanting to stay in control during my meeting with Max – I'd stuck to drinking water all evening, so I was as sober as a judge. When the train finally pulled to a halt at my stop, I hurried across the car park and clambered into my car. Sod's law being what it is, I hadn't brought my phone charger with me, but I didn't plan to ring Alex. Instead I put the car into gear, pulled out of the car park and headed for his house.

The night was dark and I was tired and anxious. I knew Alex's address, but I had never been to the village where he lived, let alone to his house. We'd always met at my place, so I wasn't exactly sure how to get there, other than in the most general sense – but how hard could it be?

Out of town, away from my familiar routes, the country roads before me twisted in and out of high hedges, picked out here and there like a ribbon in the moonlight. All the way there my mind was working overtime. What would I do if he wasn't at home? Maybe he had already set off back to the hotel where he lived while he was working away.

My imagination was causing problems again – sometimes it just jumps ship and runs wild, and when under stress it never comes up with anything very helpful or uplifting but instead goes straight for the knife drawer. Currently it was suggesting that maybe Alex, finally bored with waiting, had gone off to meet someone else or, worse, was tucked up at home in bed with someone else. After all, it would be a shame to waste his nice new flogger. It would have meant him setting someone up as a first reserve in case I went back to Max – it wasn't likely, but at that moment it felt highly likely. I felt like if I didn't see him right then and tell him how I felt, then I would lose him forever. That's romance writers for you – all melodrama and desire for a happy-ever-after!

Finally I drove into Alex's village. It was much larger than I had expected. I went through it twice before finally spotting the turning for his road. His cottage was set back from the main drag and was framed by mature trees. There was no car parked outside on the drive, no lights. It didn't look promising. The whole place was in darkness, but even so I got out, locked the car, hurried up the path and rang the doorbell. I could heard it ringing somewhere inside. I waited.

There was nothing: not a sound, not a scuffle, not so much as a whisper from inside. No light came on, nothing, which was worrying, because although it was late I knew from experience that Alex was a night owl. In my heart I knew that if he had been there he would have opened the door. *If he was alone*, my brain offered helpfully.

I rang again, holding the bell down for a little bit longer this time. There were still no sounds from inside the house. No lights. Nothing, except for the full Technicolor scenario running round inside my head, which involved Alex upstairs with someone else – someone else who he had gagged and tied to the bed, obviously.

Alex had been so patient with me, so understanding, and yet I knew damn well that if the situation had been reversed I wouldn't have been. Did Alex truly believe I was worth waiting for? And if he had changed his mind and gone off looking for someone else, how could I possibly blame him?

I stood on the doorstep getting cold, at a loss now, wondering if I should ring the doorbell one last time. Who was I kidding? If Alex hadn't heard me after two rings, another one wasn't going to make any difference. He was either out or otherwise engaged or possibly both.

All my bluster and sense of excitement evaporated, leaving me feeling deflated and miserable. Leaving Max in London and coming home, driving over to Alex's cottage in the middle of the night – let's face it, it had been a big gesture, a *Gone with the Wind* closing-credits moment, a sign that I had chosen him. And yes, of course, I could ring or come back the next day if he wasn't there tonight, but it felt like it had to be done now or never.

I wanted to show Alex that I cared enough to run away from Max and come to him, that I wanted to be with him – with *him*, and no one else – that I wanted all the things that he wanted, and that all those things about love and a life together that I hadn't let myself think about were possible with him. If I could just make him hear.

I rang one more time, letting my finger linger on the bell, even though I knew it was useless. I waited a minute or two more, just in case, and still there was nothing. Of course there wasn't. Alex quite obviously wasn't at home and I had no idea where else he might be.

I suddenly felt very alone. The night was dark and cold; the wind was whipping through the leaves. I shivered and pulled my coat tighter around me, struggling with the idea that now I had to go home without seeing him, without telling him that I had made up my mind once and for all and that he had been right all along.

Maybe Alex had already gone, driving off to his hotel and to his new contract; maybe he was out with friends; maybe – my mind busied itself knitting scenario after scenario. One thing was painfully clear: while I had been off seeing Max, Alex hadn't been sitting around at home waiting for me to ring.

After a moment or two more I sighed and turned to walk back down the path. It didn't matter how much I didn't want the evening to end this way; there was nothing else I could do. I had done my best. I wondered whether I should leave a note, but then again, if Alex was away and back at work, what difference would it make? And also him finding a note a week or more later would make me seem a bit pathetic, I felt. And what would I say? 'Hello, Alex, I was here'?

Still considering my options, I headed back down the pavement to where my car was parked under a streetlight. I was just ferreting around in my handbag looking for the keys, thinking about the long, lonely drive home, when I saw someone rounding the corner of the otherwise deserted street.

I turned and stared, concerned that my eyes might be deceiving me. But no, I was right. I would have recognised that gait anywhere. It was Alex, and as I spotted him he looked up and saw me and grinned.

My heart fluttered and I grinned too. I was so pleased to see him.

He had a bottle of wine under one arm and was carrying a takeaway bag in the other. His pace slowed as he got to me. 'Well, hello there. You're very nicely dressed for a mugger,' he said.

I nodded towards the bottle of wine and his late supper. 'Do you think there's enough there for two?' I asked.

'Why don't you come in and we'll find out,' Alex said. And with that, I followed him inside.

# Also by Sarah K

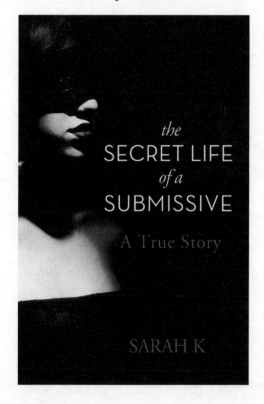

Read the first chapter now ...

# Chapter One

'I know nothing about sex
because I was always married.'
*Zsa Zsa Gabor*

'So if you could do *anything*, anything at all, what would
you do?' I asked, handing round the after-dinner mints.

Across the table, Gabbie, who is one of my oldest and
best friends, and who was busy helping herself to the last
slice of cheesecake, said, 'I'm assuming we're not talking
about hang-gliding here, are we?'

'No. In bed.'

'In bed?' said Helen. 'That restricts it a bit. How about
*out* of bed?'

'You know what I mean: if you could do anything
*sexually*.'

'Oh, you're way too coy to be a pornographer,' snorted
Gabbie.

'Do the things we've already done count?' asked Joan.

We all turned to look at her. Joan is small, lovely, and
looks like butter wouldn't melt. Back in the mists of time
she'd been a tour rep for Thomson's and up until now
what had happened on tour had most definitely stayed
on tour.

'Anything,' I repeated. 'Any time, any place, anywhere.'

'And then you're going to write about it?' said Helen, topping up her wine glass.

'Well, yes, if it's any good I will. I won't use any of your names, obviously, and I'll change it enough so that no one knows it was you.'

'That's a shame,' said Joan, taking another mint from the box. 'I'm sure Miguel and Antonio would be chuffed to bits to see their names up in lights.'

Everyone laughed. 'You're winding us up,' said Gabbie.

Joan pulled a face and then laughed. 'Oh, come on,' she said. 'We all did crazy things when we were younger.'

'I didn't,' I said, and this time it was me they all looked at. 'Well, it's true. I didn't. I was married by the time I was twenty.'

'Before then,' said Gabbie, 'you must have played around a bit.'

'I had a couple of boyfriends, but not that many. And Ray and I met when I'd just finished sixth form …' I began. 'You know that.'

Although I didn't say anything, in all the years we'd been together Ray had always preferred his sex the same way he enjoyed his food: plain, nothing fancy and without any peculiar ingredients. For him the very thought of anything that didn't involve fumbling around under the duvet with the lights off was a sign of moral turpitude, and if he had ever enjoyed it before, it wasn't the kind of thing you inflicted on your wife.

'Oh, that is classic,' snorted Helen. 'You're the one who is supposed to be writing a dirty book and you're the only one who's stuck to the straight and narrow. Fabulous.'

'It's not dirty, it's erotica, and this is exactly why I've got you lot over. So what would you do?'

We were having a fajita evening in the kitchen at Gabbie's cottage near Somerleyton.

We've been doing it for years. We used to meet up once a month when the children were smaller, but these days we get together when we can fit it into our increasingly busy lives. Every time we do it I wish we did it more.

We met at pre-natal classes in a scout hut in a little village just outside Cambridge. We've supported each other through backache, heartburn, teething, sleepless nights, terrible twos, troublesome teenagers, empty nests, dodgy marriages, cheating husbands and messy divorces. We've wept with each other, laughed with each other, got drunk with each other, and helped each other move house and move on. Remarkably we're all still friends.

Spread out over Gabbie's huge farmhouse kitchen was the debris of wrap-them-up-yourself chicken fajitas, tortilla chips, sour cream, salsa, potato wedges, white wine, Spanish beer and a big jug of margarita mix. We'd eaten our way through assorted tubs of Ben & Jerry's and a twice-baked New York cheesecake made by Joan who, after years of abstinence on the kitchen front, had started working in a cookshop, taken up the apron and turned out to be the most amazing cook.

Gabbie is a solicitor, well spoken, tall and skinny, with the most fabulous long, straight, brown hair. Whatever she's doing, she always looks as if she has just been ironed.

Helen is a gardener: strawberry blonde, ruddy complexion, capable, funny, always wears trousers or shorts and smiles a lot. There's Joan, tiny, pretty, dark-haired Joan, who manages a shop and is a deacon at her local church. And then there's me, Sarah, and I'm a writer.

I'd been writing romantic fiction for the best part of twenty years, creating modern fairy tales about handsome, flawed, lovable heroes and complex women with complicated lives, finding their way to their very own happy ever after. For the last couple of years I'd been the main breadwinner, paying the bills while my husband, Ray, went back to college full time. To make ends meet, alongside writing novels, I'd also written for magazines and newspapers, for radio, short stories, travel guides, country house handbooks – in fact anything to make a living. Which was what led a friend, another writer, to send me a newspaper clipping about a publisher that was bringing out erotic fiction specifically written for women by women. My friend suggested that we both have a go at writing something. All they wanted was three chapters and a synopsis. What had we got to lose? After all, she reasoned, the sage advice given to all writers is to write about what you know. We were both married and we knew about sex. More than that, we knew about the sex we would enjoy given half a chance, which wasn't necessarily the same as the sex we were getting.

To be frank, writing erotica had never been up there on my 'Ten things to do before I die' list, but it was a new market, I needed to earn a living and I decided it was worth a shot – after all, what was the worst that could happen? They would reject my idea. What I hadn't bargained for was that it would help change my life for ever.

You'd think writing about sex would be easy, but when, after submitting my sample chapters, I was given a commission to write my first erotic novel and started work, I discovered it isn't.

You need to find ways to describe all the bits and pieces and goings on so that it doesn't sound like a public information film; and once you get past the labelling of parts you need to make it all sound sensual and romantic, and take your reader on a slow enjoyable journey towards a rip-snorting climax.

So no pressure then.

I kept a notebook alongside my keyboard with a whole collection of stick drawings in it, a visual aid to help me to work out what you could do given time, patience and no worries about a dodgy back – man woman, woman woman, man man, twosomes, threesomes, foursomes, orgy – as well as where all the bits go. While you can more or less guess what the business end is up to, where people put their arms, knees or elbows isn't always as clear, so you need to work it out, so that the mechanics are sorted and therefore more or less invisible, and your hero won't fall over while mid-fuck.

No one in erotica *ever* falls over unless they're being swept off their feet and ravaged. They don't get cramp, or the giggles, or trip over their pants while they're trying to take them off. No one passes wind and flaps the covers, laughing furiously. Zips never get stuck, everyone always comes, and no one ever has a spotty bum. Humour and sex don't mix in erotic fiction, or so my new editor reliably informed me.

'Good erotic fiction should be like the best sex,' she said during one of our telephone conversations. 'A long, slow, satisfying build-up, hitting all the sweet spots, filling you with expectation, getting you more and more aroused, slowly bringing you closer and closer to the edge, making you gasp with pleasure, before finally taking you breathlessly to the grand finale. Erotic fiction should never let you down. Nobody in an erotic novel ever thought: let's get this over and done with, *X Factor*'s on at nine. Never, ever.'

The downside as a writer is that you need to have great sex in every chapter in lots of different, ever more exciting ways. In real life, not only is real sex not like that but also it doesn't need a plot. I'd been married a long time, and sex had long since slipped from something you were doing all the time to something squeezed into the to-do list, between cleaning out the guinea pig and collecting the kids from football practice. And unlike when you're writing about sex, during real sex you generally don't need to stop halfway through a really good bit to take the dog to the vet or nip out to buy the ingredients for your child's home economics bake-a-thon.

I hadn't got an office, so I was writing my first erotic novel on the family computer in a corner of the sitting room, squirrelling it away after each session in a desktop file labelled 'This year's tax receipts' and constantly reminding myself not to email it to my accountant. With a house full of teenagers the last thing I wanted was for them to read what I was writing, so I put an old-fashioned clothes horse around my desk, hung laundry all over it and told them it was to keep out the draught. My husband, although he knew what I was writing, never peeked. No one else in the family seemed to notice that the same towels and sheets hung there for weeks on end.

Halfway through the first book I stalled, stuttered and finally ran out of ideas. There were only so many ways our heroine could shed her clothes and gasp in breathless anticipation. Which was why Helen, Joan and I were all at Gabbie's, eating for England. They had volunteered to help me out.

'So it can be *anything?*' said Helen.

I nodded. 'Anything at all that you've ever fantasized about. Anything that you've always wanted to do, if you could do it without getting caught, and without risking disease or hurting anyone.'

'Or something we've already done,' said Gabbie, looking pointedly at Joan.

I nodded. 'I'm stuck,' I said. 'I really do need your help.'

'How tragic is that,' said Gabbie, laughing.

I was thinking they might come up with sex on a beach or in a sleeper train, or being ravished by a highwayman, but no: once they got going and were halfway through the Baileys, they were swapping real-life sexploits.

One had had sex on a cross-Channel ferry in the 1970s with a Frenchman she picked up in Duty Free, and when he told her that he wanted to see her again and asked for her name and telephone number, she lied through her teeth and told him her name was Freda and that she came from Margate.

Another had had a three-in-a-bed session with two builders who came to fix her parents' roof when she had been home from college in her twenties. Another admitted to a drunken lesbian romp while on a painting holiday in Tuscany – as she said, it wasn't something she particularly wanted to do again but she was glad she'd tried it. Which really did make it sound a bit like abseiling or hang-gliding – but she did add that it was incredibly refreshing to have sex with someone who actually knew where all your bits were.

I made notes – lots of notes.

'Oh, and then I went out with this guy, after I split up with Keith. Do you remember Stuart?' asked Gabbie. 'Big, sort of gingery?' She mimed tall with hair.

We all nodded.

'He used to like to spank me.'

I stared at her. 'And did you like it?'

Gabbie shrugged in a non-committal way. 'It was OK, I suppose. I think he was hoping it would turn me on, but it didn't. He kept saying that he'd really like to tie me up.'

'Oh, we tried that,' said Helen. 'The kids were at my mum's for the weekend. We did the whole thing: candlelit dinner, sexy underwear, silk scarf for a blindfold. Gav in this silk bathrobe I'd bought him for his birthday.' Helen grinned. 'God, I mean, he spent hours. It was fabulous. The only trouble was I wriggled so much that he couldn't get the bloody knots undone when we'd finished and had to cut me off the bed with a pair of scissors. I'd got a blindfold on, so it wasn't until he took it off I realized he'd used Molly's skipping rope. God, she was livid.'

'I blame *Cosmopolitan*,' said Gabbie, sucking chocolate out of her teeth.

'I've always fancied doing that,' I said, casually. 'Being tied up.'

'You should suggest it to Ray,' said Joan. 'Lots of men get off on that kind of thing. You know: helpless virgin, tied to a bed.' She rolled her eyes and waved her hands, squealing, 'Help, help,' in a very passable impression of Penelope Pitstop.

What I didn't tell them, and had never really admitted to myself until then, was that I'd fantasized about being tied up and spanked for years: not all the time, obviously, and it wasn't my only sexual fantasy, but it was there, carefully hidden and tucked at the back of my mind, and it was something I constantly revisited. The idea was a huge turn-on and had been for as long as I could remember – certainly long before my thoughts had turned to sex.

When it came to playing cowboys and Indians as a child, I had been the one who always volunteered to be held captive and tied to a tree. Want someone to hold hostage or whip until they give up the whereabouts of the cowboy encampment? Oooooo, oooo, yes please, that'd be me.

As I got older the fantasies became more explicit, and eventually sexual, and evolved to being put over someone's knee and soundly spanked, or being whipped with a riding crop, tied up or down, and made to do all sorts of interesting naughty things that my mother never told me about and certainly wouldn't approve of. But in all that time I had always kept these thoughts to myself. There was a part of me that was afraid to admit how much the idea excited me.

'Bob used to like me to tie him up,' said Joan conversationally, 'and thrash him with the cane on the feather duster. It wasn't really my kind of thing but he liked it. I used to find the feather duster upstairs in the bathroom and think: Oh, here we go again. He bought me a French maid's outfit the Christmas before we split ...'

In my fantasies the someone who did those wonderful things to me was always a broad-shouldered, dashingly handsome Prince Charming, who was good-looking in a clean-cut preppy kind of a way, and who was totally in control. He didn't say very much because, as is the way with fantasies, he always knew exactly what I wanted and when I wanted it, and was terribly good at giving it to me right on cue.

I'd be wearing high heels and I'd squeal in a girlie way, and after he had spanked me he would carry me over to a big four-poster bed and tie me down and blindfold me, before going to work with his knowing fingers and even more knowing tongue; then, when I was baying for more, he would make love to me, long and slow, until we both finally came. Visually it was a treat of rich colours, soft leather, huge four-poster beds, hairy chests and muscular torsos, and it was a fantasy that I kept on having, as I reworked the details.

I'd never told anyone about wanting to be spanked or whipped or tied down, because I was pretty much convinced that I was alone in thinking those kinds of things and finding a sexual charge in them. I assumed that they were definitely too weird to talk about, and certainly way too weird to do anything about. Yet here were my best friends talking about exactly that. Maybe what I wanted wasn't that unusual after all.

As I'd been taking notes, I was the only one who hadn't had a drink, and I drove home thinking through what the girls had told me. Looking in through the sitting-room window, I could see Ray slumped on the sofa watching TV in his tracksuit bottoms and a T-shirt. We'd been together for a long time; we had kids, dogs and a home together. Things weren't great between us. Money was tight, and while I was working every hour I could to try to keep our noses above water (he had been made redundant in a departmental rationalization and was now back at college, retraining), he refused to help by even thinking about a part-time job or helping round the house. As far as he was concerned, all that, and the children, were my responsibility, whether he was working or not. I was tired in lots of ways.

If you asked him, Ray would tell you with some pride that he was an old-fashioned man – a man who liked his wife at home. A proper family was what he called it. He'd probably have had a heart attack if I'd mentioned the whole tying-up thing. He was, and still is, a very practical man, a careful man; for him romance, luxury and adventurous sex were things other people had and I'd always felt he rather despised them.

As I unlocked the front door I thought about what Gabbie had said about sharing my fantasies with him, and realized with a growing certainty that it was probably too late.

Ray didn't even look away from the TV as I slipped off my coat. 'How did it go?' he asked.

'Oh, OK. I just want to get some of these notes down before I forget them,' I said.

He nodded, eyes still firmly fixed on the TV screen. With a sigh, I walked over to the computer, turned it on and got to work.

Over the next few weeks in every spare moment I worked on my first erotic novel. I reworked my friends' adventures and wove in all the things that turned me on. And more and more I had a sense of escaping into a fantasy world where anything was possible. I started to write all those things that had fuelled my fantasies for so long – and it was heady stuff. Most of them revolved around a tall, dark, handsome older man, who took control, and understood the heroine and what she needed and wanted, and gave them without question – with unconditional love and understanding. He was my Prince Charming, the alpha man of my fantasies.

I wondered, as I wrote, if that was what I thought I'd seen in Ray when I first met him. He was fifteen years older than me; I'd been working in a hotel for the summer when he asked me out. I'd seen him as capable, strong and silent. Things that at eighteen I had naïvely taken as positive qualities had, over the years, revealed themselves to be altogether less positive, and traits that probably a woman of his own age would have instantly recognized. He was stubborn and uncommunicative, and had, I suspected, chosen a much younger wife so that he could try to mould her into the woman he wanted. We got along fine until I wanted to grow up and have a life of my own.

Although I hadn't anticipated it, writing erotica was the perfect escape from the realities of a crumbling marriage. All those things that I'd never told anyone before, all those things I had longed to explore, finally had a place and a purpose.

I also spent a lot of time doing research on the internet, which up until that point I'd mostly used to buy shoes and books. Not altogether sure what I'd find, I was nervous, excited, sometimes shocked and sometimes delighted. The internet opened up a whole new world. I rapidly discovered that far from my being alone in my fantasies there was a whole sub-culture out there that I had known nothing about, and lots and lots of people who felt the same as I did. I wasn't so much relieved as stunned. And even better was that I found I had a name: I was a submissive.

In my fantasies, at least, I was a submissive – the one who gets spanked and tied up and gets all the attention. *Submissive*. I certainly didn't see myself as submissive in real life, but sexually I could see that it was a good fit.

Having sold my first attempt at writing female erotica, I wrote more – a lot more. The stuff that had fuelled my fantasies for years was suddenly fuelling my fiction and my finances; and having finally found a home for all those things I'd been dreaming about since my teens felt good. Having an outlet for my innermost thoughts helped paper over the cracks in my increasingly unhappy marriage, and I was having the best sex of my life, albeit on the page.

Over the next five years I wrote twelve novels and countless short stories. The books and short stories always involved some degree of bondage and submission, and other sexual shenanigans that can be loosely described as S&M (sadism and masochism) and BDSM (bondage, discipline, sadism and masochism), but in all that time, as I was writing about it and fantasizing about it, I never once tried any of it – not one single glorious black-leather, high-heeled, handcuffed moment of it. And Ray never read my books. Not one, ever.

Books, as Ray was eager to point out to anyone who would listen, were not his thing – and eventually, neither was I.

Finally the cracks just got too big and we separated. We were divorced within a year. It took me a while to get myself together, but after a few months I started, very tentatively, to date again. Fresh out of a long-term relationship, I wasn't altogether sure exactly how or where to begin. So after a few false starts I turned to the place where a lot of us begin again: internet dating websites.

I think we're often drawn to various incarnations of the devil we know – a type – and, having been married a long time, I certainly was. The men I dated after leaving Ray all seemed to have been cut from the same cloth. I was obviously doing something wrong. The men were all steady and practical, and I was still having married sex; I was just having it with new men.

Then along came Henry, my first attempt at trying to combine what passes for normal with some of the things I'd been fantasizing about.

After two glasses of house red and a light supper on our first weekend away together, I asked Henry if he'd ever thought about spanking anyone. You know – for fun. His eyes widened and his face took on an expression similar to the one I'd last seen on the face of a woman I'd offered a bacon butty, seconds before discovering she was a hard-line vegan.

Henry visibly stiffened and said, all outrage and horror, 'Good Lord, certainly not! What on earth do you think I am – some kind of a pervert?'

Well, yes, hopefully.

'Don't you have any fantasies?' I pressed, emboldened by strong drink and a nasty sinking feeling. The relation-ship had been pretty much doomed since lunchtime, when we'd been about to go Dutch on an uninspiring quiche and green salad when Henry had pointed out that actually I'd had a cappuccino and a sweet.

'Of course I have fantasies,' he said, 'but mostly they involve world peace and captaining the English cricket team during a one-day test at Headingley.'

Buddhists, what can I tell you?

So how did he feel about underwear? What sort of thing did he like? I asked, giving it one last shot and my voice dropping to a seductive purr.

'I haven't given it a lot of thought, to be perfectly honest.' He paused and then said, 'Something from Marks, probably.' I watched him slipping a bread roll into his pocket in case he got a bit peckish later. It wasn't the answer I'd hoped for, to be honest.

So that was it: I was a pervert. My first very tentative attempt at expressing what I wanted – fuelled by a little wine and a lot of nerve – had been thrown back in my face. It confirmed what I had feared: nice men didn't find this kind of stuff acceptable.

It was during that weekend that I decided it was time I found some way to let the genie out of the bottle and go in search of something else – something a little more rock and roll. I was in my mid-forties with a broken marriage and three children in their late teens and early twenties, and I wanted to try some of those things I had always dreamed of and been writing about, before it was too late. What had I got to lose?

It's a scary journey to start all on your own. What I needed was a guide: someone to help me find my way through a sexual landscape about which, despite several books, in reality I had absolutely no idea – and more to the point, someone who I felt I could trust enough to bring me out wiser but unscathed on the other side.

It had also occurred to me that maybe when I got to the point of experimenting I would chicken out, so I also needed someone with a sense of humour and a lot of patience: someone who wouldn't freak out if ultimately I put it all down to research.

I'm not sure I was setting out on a journey to look for a

happy-ever-after with anyone, but there definitely had to be a spark, that magic indefinable something between us. What I needed was a hero, a dominant man – referred to as a Dom in the BDSM world – who I could trust implicitly and who I liked, and who was prepared to help me, and spank me, and who I fancied. And we all know how very easy men like that are to find …

Then again, if I didn't try now, my fantasies would stay just that and I might as well settle down with someone like Henry and look forward to a lifetime of sensible pants and going Dutch.

When I arrived home after our weekend away I dumped him, put 'BDSM' into a search engine and watched the hits roll in. It is astonishing what you can find if you ask the right questions. There is everything you can ever want on the net and much more besides. Some of it in leather, some in plus sizes and an awful lot of it in America.

As I stared at the screen, flicking between websites, it occurred to me that I really needed to work out exactly what it was I was looking for. As research projects go I've had far worse. I made a list.